RACIAL TRAUMA IN BLACK CLIENTS

RACIAL TRAUMA in Black Clients

Effective Practice for Clinicians

Jennifer R. Jones-Damis
Kelly N. Moore

Foreword by Nancy Boyd-Franklin

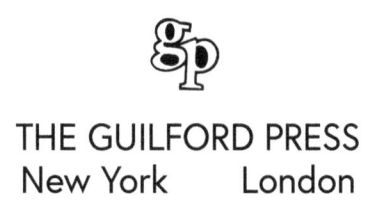

THE GUILFORD PRESS
New York   London

Copyright © 2025 The Guilford Press
A Division of Guilford Publications, Inc.
www.guilford.com

All rights reserved

No part of this book may be reproduced, translated, stored in a retrieval system, or transmitted, in any form or by any means, electronic, mechanical, photocopying, microfilming, recording, or otherwise, without written permission from the publisher.

Printed in the United States of America

This book is printed on acid-free paper.

The authors have checked with sources believed to be reliable in their efforts to provide information that is complete and generally in accord with the standards of practice that are accepted at the time of publication. However, in view of the possibility of human error or changes in behavioral, mental health, or medical sciences, neither the authors, nor the editors and publisher, nor any other party who has been involved in the preparation or publication of this work warrants that the information contained herein is in every respect accurate or complete, and they are not responsible for any errors or omissions or the results obtained from the use of such information. Readers are encouraged to confirm the information contained in this book with other sources.

Last digit is print number: 9 8 7 6 5 4 3 2 1

Library of Congress Cataloging-in-Publication Data is available from the publisher.

ISBN 978-1-4625-5659-5 (paperback)
ISBN 978-1-4625-5693-9 (cloth)

I am truly blessed by God to have an amazingly supportive husband, Jean-Frederic, who helped me bring three miracles into the world, my children, Justice, Jericho, and Jade. They are the driving force behind my desire to make this world a better place. I am forever grateful to my parents, Linda McQuilla-Jones and Barry Jones, who instilled in me a desire to do right in this world and to continue to pave a path for future generations. Thank you to my sister, Vanessa Nedrick, her husband, Jason Nedrick Sr., and their two beautiful sons, Jason Jr. and Jordan, for being a constant reminder of what Black Love truly is and can be. Finally, to my church family at Second Baptist Church of Roselle, New Jersey, my entire family, and my dear friends, thank you for your support during my professional and personal journey in life. I love you and thank you all for being a part of my village. To the clinicians who are ready to do the much-needed work inside of these pages, thank you for going on this journey with us. Here we go!

—JENNIFER R. JONES-DAMIS

I dedicate this book to the people who have been in my corner, always propelling me to be my best and encouraging me through prayer, love, and support in every way. To my incredibly supportive husband, Melvin—thank you for believing in me and always remaining steady and prayerful for us. To our three amazing boys—Miles, Mason, and Matthew—thank you for being a necessary and welcome reminder of what #BlackBoyJoy looks like. I also dedicate this book to my parents, Michael and Diana Walker. Mom—I know you are looking down on me and always protecting me. Your life as a social worker and advocate for children laid the foundation for the work I do now. I love and miss you every day. Dad—thank you for every word of encouragement and your ever-present humor to help me keep things in perspective. To my sister, Kimberly—thank you for being the best sister anyone could ask for! To all those whom I get the privilege to call my family and friends—thank you for being a part of my village, for your prayers, and constant love. And finally, I dedicate this book to all the Black mothers and fathers who have lost loved ones to race-based violence. You are not forgotten, and we know our work must continue in whatever lane we occupy to shine a light on racial violence and its impact on those we work with.

—KELLY N. MOORE

About the Authors

Jennifer R. Jones-Damis, PsyD, is Director of the Counseling Center at Rutgers, The State University of New Jersey. She is an active participant with the National Child Traumatic Stress Network (NCTSN), particularly on the Schools Committee and the Justice Consortium Committee. Dr. Jones-Damis's research interests focus on understanding and addressing traumatic stress and racial trauma in individuals and systems. She holds positions on the state and national boards of the Association of Black Psychologists.

Kelly N. Moore, PsyD, is Director of the Center for Psychological Services in the Graduate School of Applied and Professional Psychology at Rutgers, The State University of New Jersey. She also has a private practice providing mental health treatment, training, and consultation. Dr. Moore's clinical foci are trauma, anxiety, and perinatal disorders, and she consults and trains professionals and graduate students on culturally responsive supervision, racial trauma, and the influence of culture on the manifestation of mental health challenges.

Foreword

Trauma and complex trauma have become central topics in the mental health field in recent years. Many clinicians who pride themselves on providing trauma-informed care have had no training in the reality of racial trauma in the lives of many of their Black clients. Racial trauma or race-based traumatic stress (Carter, 2007) is complex and may be attributable to varied experiences and sources of racism and discrimination that impact an African American individual's mental and physical health (Comas-Díaz, Hall, & Neville, 2019). Racial trauma may result from a single incident of an overwhelming nature that includes danger or the threat of injury or death. It may also result from the cumulative effects, throughout a Black person's life, of multiple experiences of derogatory statements, disrespect, humiliating or shaming events, racial microaggressions, as well as other overt examples of racism and discrimination.

Racial trauma may also be experienced vicariously. Vicarious racial trauma has a long history in the lives of African Americans. During slavery, Black individuals were often forced to be present as acts of brutality were inflicted on their own people. Today, advances in technology have made the impact of vicarious racial trauma even more widespread. It is commonplace for cell phone videos of the murder of African Americans to be shown repeatedly on television and disseminated widely on social media. Witnessing harmful and/or painful incidents, such as repeated viewings of brutality, shootings, and killings perpetrated against members of one's racial group, can elicit feelings of fear for oneself as well as for one's partners, children, grandchildren, and other family members (Helms, Nicolas, & Green, 2012).

Although racial trauma has been part of the academic literature for many years, it was not until the murder of George Floyd, a Black man, by a white police officer in May of 2020 that it became a more familiar term to many clinicians. In the years since his death, when I have given trainings on racial trauma throughout the United States and abroad, I have been surprised by the number of clinicians who have never heard the term. They recall their own shock when they saw George Floyd killed before their eyes on their TVs or on social media, but it is still difficult for many therapists to find the words to ask their Black clients about racism and the vicarious racial trauma they may have experienced when they witnessed this devastating event and others like it. Many clinicians, particularly those from other cultural groups, were hesitant to raise these issues for fear of offending their clients. This was compounded by the fact that many Black people may not be familiar with the expression "racial trauma," a clinical and psychological term. Many clinicians did not realize that the avoidance of these issues might retraumatize their Black clients and increase the suspicion they may feel toward therapy.

The murder of George Floyd was a major tragic event for individuals of many backgrounds throughout the world. For numerous African Americans, however, there has been a seemingly endless number of Black men and women who have been killed throughout their lives. Many African Americans remember the names of Eric Garner, Breonna Taylor, Philando Castile, Michael Brown, and many other Black men and women who have been killed by the police. For Black parents and grandparents, intense fear for their children can be triggered by memories of the shooting of Tamir Rice, a 12-year-old Black boy killed by the police while playing outside a playground with a toy gun in Cleveland, Ohio. This fear was also triggered by the murder of Trayvon Martin, a 17-year-old Black adolescent who was walking home from a convenience store when he was killed by George Zimmerman, a member of the neighborhood watch in a gated community in Florida. Given these realities, it is important for clinicians to remember that each of these experiences can trigger fear, anger, rage, a sense of loss, a sense of helplessness, and racial trauma for many African Americans.

After incidents such as these, clinicians may work with African American parents who are struggling with intense fear for their children and feel the need to provide racial socialization in order to prepare them for experiences of racism, without making them bitter or negative in their approach to the world. I remember vividly, after the death of George Floyd, a number of therapists who see primarily adults in individual therapy contacted me for advice when their Black clients asked for help in the struggle to talk to their children about this incident and about race, racism, and racial trauma. This book provides clinicians, particularly those from other cultures, with unique insights into the multigenerational use of racial socialization by Black families to empower their children and to help them develop a strong sense of racial identity to inoculate them against the effects of racism. Since slavery, Black families have utilized a number of important strategies, including "The Talk" about racism, to strengthen their children and prepare them for these experiences. This book discusses myriad ways in which clinicians can utilize these strategies in therapy to help Black parents discuss such issues with their children.

Throughout my experience of over 45 years as a therapist, supervisor, professor, and trainer, I have worked with many African American clinicians who have experienced racial trauma during their training in university programs, in their workplaces, and in the broader mental health field. While clinicians may be responsive to the racial trauma that their clients experience, they often do not recognize that their Black colleagues also contend with race-based traumatic stress and racial trauma. As Black people, these clinicians additionally experience ongoing occurrences of racism, discrimination, microaggressions, slights, insults, and lack of respect. Sadly, many of these incidents are the result of interactions with their professors, fellow students or colleagues, and supervisors. In addition, for many Black mental health providers, viewing repeated images of Black people being killed or brutalized, and listening to clients of the same background reporting experiences of racial trauma, can increase their own traumatic response—a process captured by the notion of vicarious racial trauma. Jennifer R. Jones-Damis and Kelly N. Moore have made a major contribution by bringing this "compounding" effect to our attention and offering ways in which we can support our Black colleagues and recognize the burdens they may carry in responding to their own racial trauma as well as that of their clients. In addition, the authors emphasize that it is important to acknowledge and address Black colleagues' actions by other mental health professionals that might contribute to their racial trauma; provide culturally sensitive therapy; and encourage self-care during these difficult periods.

Jones-Damis and Moore also offer clinicians an important analysis of the influence that various systems may have in their Black clients' lives, a subject often overlooked in many training programs. This oversight is particularly problematic when working with Black clients who must contend with individual as well as systemic or institutional racism. Therapists may find themselves working with clients who encounter racism within the school system or in community settings. With this in mind, these authors have given us an insightful view of the types of racial trauma that Black children may experience from their early years through their adolescence in school systems across the country. Their discussion of the "school-to-prison pipeline" is particularly powerful. Clinicians within the school system (e.g., guidance counselors, school counselors, social workers, and school psychologists) are in a unique position to intervene in the lives of these children and their parents, and to provide intervention and mediation for them.

African American culture is collectivistic. As a result, when an incident of racism and racial trauma occurs, the impact is not limited to individuals in the community where the event took place. For example, in 2015, nine individuals attending a bible study in a Black church in Charleston, South Carolina, were killed by a white man. The shock and vicarious racial trauma of this incident were felt in Black churches and communities across the country. Although many therapists wanted to help these congregations, they often lacked the training necessary to engage successfully in culturally competent community interventions. Jones-Damis and Moore draw on Afrocentric group interventions to describe ways in which these skills can be utilized to address racial trauma in Black communities after this type of incident.

Many clinicians, particularly those from other racial and ethnic groups, have been searching for a book that will help them address the issues of race, racism, and racial trauma in therapy with Black clients. The vivid case examples and clear dialogues in this book provide a roadmap for discussing these issues with openness and cultural humility. The authors illustrate the ways in which utilizing cultural humility in therapy can build trust with African American clients. In addition, this book will make an outstanding contribution to the mental health field by opening the eyes of clinicians to the many ways in which racial trauma can affect their Black clients. Therapists of all backgrounds will benefit from the illustrations of how therapists can initiate these discussions and incorporate them into therapy, as a response to both direct experiences of racism and vicarious racial trauma. This approach will help clinicians form strong therapeutic alliances with their Black clients and empower them to heal from the effects of racial trauma in their lives.

NANCY BOYD-FRANKLIN, PhD
Author of *Black Families in Therapy:
Understanding the African American Experience*

References

Carter, R. (2007). Racism and psychological and emotional injury: Recognizing and assessing race-based traumatic stress. *The Counseling Psychologist*, 35(1), 13–105.

Comas-Díaz, L., Hall, G. N., & Neville, H. (2019). Racial trauma: Theory, research, and healing: Introduction to the Special Issue. *American Psychologist*, 74(1), 1–5.

Helms, J., Nicolas, G., & Green, C. (2012). Racism and ethnoviolence as trauma: Enhancing professional and research training. *Traumatology*, 18(1), 65–74.

Preface

> Over and above the political, economic, sociological, and international implications of racial prejudices, their major significance is that they place unnecessary burdens upon human beings.
> —Kenneth Clark

In 2020, George Floyd was murdered by a police officer in broad daylight, and the video footage was captured and shared millions of times, reaching an international audience. This happened amid a historic global pandemic, which resulted in billions of people across the globe being quarantined and tuning in to social media and news coverage in unprecedented numbers. What happened after that sparked a prominent discussion that has always existed in the homes and communities of Black people, but now was visible in a way that felt uniquely seismic. Coupled with the increased focus on managing mental health during such challenging times, the sociocultural landscape was primed to have a more honest and challenging discussion about the intersection of race, trauma, and mental health.

Where does racism fit into this discussion about trauma and mental health?

The real question is, where *doesn't* it?

Racism is a system. To reduce it to describing a person and their actions diminishes how far-reaching and insidious the system is. Racism hides in plain sight in many forms. As clinicians, it is imperative that we understand how racism is the groundwater that gives life to the circumstances, systems, and environments that can lead to the elevated risks of trauma in Black clients. If we are truly culturally responsive, trauma-informed clinicians, we have to understand racial trauma and how it shows up in those we serve, in those we supervise, and even within ourselves.

This book is for therapists who wish to better help Black clients by understanding the ever-present nature of racism and its impact on their daily lives. Additionally, we aim to challenge therapists to approach, rather than avoid, conversations with their clients about racism, discrimination, and the toxic stress these experiences can cause for Black individuals and communities. We also aim to challenge therapists to consider the influential role they can play within traditional therapy rooms, but also in the role of consultant, trainer, or support in community settings—as well as in their professional work within systems that have historically perpetuated oppressive practices and policies that disenfranchise Black people.

In Part I, we discuss research on trauma and adverse childhood experience in an effort to support the idea that systemic racism can be a toxic stressor for Black clients. And we offer strategies for how to apply this knowledge in traditional clinical settings.

In Part II, we discuss the impact of racial trauma in community settings and how therapists can integrate awareness of community systems to aid Black clients in coping with racism-based stressors. These chapters focus on working with youth in school settings, with law enforcement, and with parents helping their children navigate racial prejudice and biases.

Finally, Part III focuses on the importance of self-care for therapists who engage in the work of creating brave spaces to help clients process and cope with racial trauma. Helping professionals need to recognize and head off their own risks for vicarious trauma and compassion fatigue. We offer ideas not only on how to help clients heal, but also on recognizing oneself as a healer in need of preservation to prevent the occupational hazard of burnout.

Throughout the text, there are bolded terms defined in the Glossary at the back of the book. We know that the work of understanding racial trauma is ever-evolving, and no list of terms is comprehensive, but we aimed to ensure that the Glossary included key terms and phrases that will provide the reader with easy guidance to understand the information shared throughout the chapters.

The terms "African American" and "Black" are intentionally used throughout this book to describe clients and summarize research findings. In situations where composite patient examples are given, we use the term that the client or family identified as, and for summaries of research studies with specific use of either term, we apply what the authors of those studies used. Elsewhere in the book, we use the term "Black" to signify that discrimination and bias are experienced by Black people, regardless of their ethnicity (e.g., African American, Caribbean American, African). But we also understand and highlight that there are some aspects of the experiences of African American families and clients that are unique.

We have also used the pronouns "they" and "them" in instances where a subject's gender is not specific or self-identified by the composite case clients.

We hope this book serves as a primer to take a deeper dive into the topic of racial trauma in Black clients. While no singular text can capture all aspects of such a robust topic that impacts many people whom clinicians encounter, we hope that this text, used in tandem with additional literature referenced throughout, will improve clinicians' understanding of racial trauma and the systems that perpetuate it, contributing to stress, anxiety, and other emotional health challenges in Black clients. The convergence of the COVID-19 pandemic, the resurgence of the Black Lives Matter movement, and diminished stigma regarding mental health treatment seeking provide an opportunity to expand our views and scopes of practice to meet the needs of Black clients in a trauma-informed and culturally humble manner.

Acknowledgments

There are many who have contributed to the development and completion of this book. We must first thank and acknowledge the mentorship and support of Dr. Nancy Boyd-Franklin. Thank you for unselfishly sharing your professional and personal advice, talent, and resources with us as your former students. This book would not have come to fruition without your guidance and pep talks!

Thank you to the pioneers in this work on the impact of racism and trauma on the lives of Black Americans. Drs. Joy DeGruy, Kenneth Hardy, Riana Elyse Anderson, Howard Stevenson, Cheryl Tawede Grills, and countless other renowned researchers and writers have provided amazing resources that paved the way for us to discuss the topic of race-based traumatic stress. We acknowledge and pay homage to their great works and contributions to our field.

Thank you to our Rutgers colleagues—past and present—who offered their support in our efforts to bring this work to life: Kaitlin Gonzales-Swanson, Kirby Wycoff, Schenike Massie-Lambert, Shalonda Kelly, Anne Gregory, and the late Pauline Hines. Your support, collaboration, and instruction gave us a strong foundation on which we have been able to build careers that afforded us real-world understanding of the tremendous impact of racism on the mental health of Black clients.

Special thanks to the Association of Black Psychologists and the New Jersey Psychological Association, whose members nurtured us throughout our academic and professional careers. It was within these organizations that our passion to liberate Black minds through psychology and our writings emerged, and for that we will forever be grateful.

Contents

PART I. RACIAL TRAUMA IN CLINICAL SETTINGS

1. Where Do We Begin?: Racial Trauma and Thinking Beyond Diagnosis — 3

2. Thinking Outside the Box: Treatment Adaptations to Address Racial Trauma — 16

3. Awareness in Action: Understanding the Barriers and Facilitators to Treatment Seeking — 32

4. Preparing the Next Generation: Culturally Responsive Supervision — 43

PART II. RACIAL TRAUMA IN COMMUNITY SETTINGS

5. Pen or Pencil: Addressing Racial Trauma in Schools — 63

6. Black and Blue: Working with Law Enforcement — 85

7. The Talk: Helping Parents and Children with Racial Traumas	105

PART III. HEALING FROM RACIAL TRAUMA

8. Healer, Heal Me: Healing Clients from Racial Trauma	127
9. Healer, Heal Thyself: Vicarious Racial Trauma and Self-Care	145
Conclusion: Summing It All Up	159
Glossary	163
References	169
Index	181

PART I

RACIAL TRAUMA IN CLINICAL SETTINGS

CHAPTER 1

Where Do We Begin?
Racial Trauma and Thinking Beyond Diagnosis

> Black folks come from a history where a woman would be forced to watch as her own child was sold and sent to an unknown place never to be seen again and told to quit crying or get beaten and return to work in the field as if nothing ever happened! Our ability to recover may seem like "natural resilience," but it's resilience born out of our ability to grieve being snuffed out. The only acceptable response to terror was to just . . . recover and get back to IT . . . whatever IT was. And it was taught over and over again.
> —MICHAEL, age 70

Sean, a 17-year-old young Black man picks up his phone and sees a text message from his best friend. It reads, "DID YOU SEE THIS?!" Included in the text message is a link that leads Sean to a video of the George Floyd incident. Sean's heart rate starts to go up. He feels his face warming up. He keeps watching. He's seen several videos like this before, but this one feels weird. It's . . . long. He keeps watching, all the way to the end. While watching, Sean mutters his thoughts out loud, even though he is in his bedroom watching alone. "Why does this keep happening? They can just kill us in broad daylight." He feels a lump in his throat. He takes a deep breath and shakes his head. Then he grips his phone and sits still for a moment. Suddenly, Sean throws the phone across the room and screams an obscenity so loud, his mother runs in to ask what is going on.

Two weeks later, while driving home from school, Sean hears a police siren. He checks his rearview mirror and sees he's being pulled over. Sean doesn't notice it, but he grips the steering wheel with both hands, his heart rate increases, and he starts to feel nervous. He glances at his phone. "Should I pick it up and call someone or record?," he thinks. The officer taps on the window, abruptly making Sean realize he never pulled down his window. "Son, do you know why I stopped you?" Sean just stares. He's sweating a little now, but he can't tell if the officer notices. "No, officer." "Where are you coming from?," the officer asks. Sean looks up nervously and then glances back at his cell phone in the passenger seat. He can't grab it now to record or call anyone. Too late. He answers back, "From school. I live right around this corner." The officer looks at him for a moment. Sean feels as if he could faint from the amount of tension in his body right now. "OK," the officer says," I stopped you because this is a school zone, and you were driving a little too fast. Slow it down. I will let you go since you are so close to home." The officer walks off. Sean leans back in the driver's seat. He puts his hands to his face and can feel the sweat. He drives home thinking, "I could have never seen my mom again. . . ."

Years later, Sean, now 24 years old, has come to your office reporting that he always feels anxious. He doesn't trust work colleagues, has racing thoughts that lead to sleepless nights, struggles with perfectionism at work, and generally never feels "settled." Sean denies any family history of anxiety, depression, or other mental health issues and currently lives alone and works in a corporate setting. He presents with a calm demeanor, makes eye contact, and takes time to ponder his words prior to answering your questions. When you ask about any history of a traumatic experience, Sean says he can't think of anything significant.

When clients enter treatment, as clinicians, we use what they tell us their presenting issue is and ask questions or offer measures to ascertain a deeper understanding of what challenges they are facing, in order to come up with a strategy to treat them. If a client comes in expressing that anxiety is their current major stressor, we tend to use that as an entry point to take a deeper dive to better understand how it affects their life and figure out a plan. What if a client has a hard time articulating what exactly is going on? In Sean's case, where would you even begin if he does not seem to have a sense of where this anxiety is coming from? Would you know what to ask him?

Much has been written in academic literature about the impact of **trauma** on brain development and long-term health, and about the way those impacted learn how to survive in the world. Research has found that early and chronic exposure to adverse childhood experience and adverse community environments can lead to tremendous stress, hypervigilance, and overall distressing thoughts and feelings about oneself and others. Repeated exposure to stress and trauma results in a person's vigilance for spotting threat becoming overactive, triggering the body's stress response (think: fight-or-flight response) so often that it becomes the default response to stressors of any magnitude (Felitti et al., 1998; Harris, 2018; Dye, 2018; Cronholm et al., 2015; Winfrey & Perry, 2021). This extra sensitivity to threat is not an indication that a person is broken or doing anything wrong. They have simply adapted to a world that puts them in situations where the risk of not being ready for threat is high. In the words of one of our adolescent clients, "I stay ready so I never have to GET ready." "Staying ready" is a natural and adaptive response to an environment that feels unpredictably yet chronically unsafe or threatening. The short-term benefit is the perceived feeling of control and preparation, but being in a constant state of readiness has both psychological and physiological impact.

Staying ready has hidden and long-term health risks. These include anxiety, fear, social withdrawal, depressed mood, avoidance, and even substance use to cope with the feelings of any of these symptoms. Some other ways chronic stress exposure can show up is in a person's trying to "disappear" to avoid being targeted, or to behave and be perfect so they will not be attacked. Consider the example of Sean. He is describing anxiety, isolation and lack of trust with colleagues, perfectionism, and feeling on edge. For clinicians who want to better understand the impact of racism in the lives of Black clients and how it relates to trauma, it is critical to have foundational knowledge of what is known about trauma, **toxic stress**, and their links to racism in America.

Trauma, Toxic Stress, and Neurobiological Impact

In 1998, the Adverse Childhood Experiences (ACE) Study was published. Based on many accounts, it was received unceremoniously by professionals in the medical field (Burke-Harris, 2018). Physicians were reticent to adopt the idea that medical health outcomes were connected to social or psychological experiences from a patient's life. The study origins are based in an observation that Vincent Felitti made in a weight-loss program he was running in his lab. Successful weight-loss patients who later gained their weight back attributed this weight gain to reasons rooted in social and psychological factors (e.g., weight being a protective factor to ward off sexual assault was reported by one of the patients). The original ACE study (Felitti et al., 1998) was born when Felitti presented his initial hunch regarding the relationship between poor health outcomes and early childhood adversity. He partnered with colleagues from the Centers for Disease Control (CDC) to conduct this groundbreaking epidemiological study. Although it took over a decade for the ACE study to gain much attention, the findings from it were fairly astounding, indicating a high dose–response relationship between early exposure to adversity and adulthood illnesses and conditions that were tied to some of the top causes of early death in adulthood. In the original ACE study, 10 items were identified as ACEs, including situations like living with a parent with mental illness, growing up with a parent who physically or sexually abused you, and witnessing domestic violence. The sample was overwhelmingly white and mostly male, but yielded remarkable results that led to subsequent research expanding on the initial study (Felitti et al., 1998).

One of these subsequent research studies—the Philadelphia Urban ACE Survey (2012–2013)—examined the methodology of the ACE study, while adding potential stressors to the original 10 items in an effort to explore the impact of racism, witnessing violence, and living in neighborhoods that respondents identified as unsafe. The sample reflected more diversity in terms of race and gender identity of the respondents. Overall, the Philadelphia ACE study revealed that not only were respondents endorsing ACEs at a higher rate, but also they had higher rates of the downstream illnesses mentioned above, compared to those in the original ACE study. The findings of the Philadelphia Urban ACE Survey indicated the need for services that not only address the *interpersonal* adversity but the *environmental stressors* that exacerbate poor health outcomes for youth and adults seeking care. Philadelphia had a population of 1.2 million people at the time of the survey. It was diverse in terms of race and education, thus making it an ideal population to expound on the work done in the original ACE study. It also helped to contribute to making the case for what we now often refer to as "social determinants of health" because it included environmental stressors such as racism as adverse childhood experiences.

Psychological trauma is often described as an experience or collection of experiences that overwhelms a person's sense of control over their life, resulting in extreme stress, vulnerability, and lack of predictability, leading to an inability to experience a sense of *felt* safety (Blaustein & Kinniburgh, 2018). The terms **complex trauma** and **psychological trauma** are used interchangeably in some literature. Scholars in the field of traumatic stress research have often encouraged clinicians to take the approach with clients that comes from the place of asking, "What *happened* to you?" as opposed to "What is *wrong* with you?" If we embrace this clinical approach to care, then we cannot deny in good faith that the way people are treated can have an impact on their *felt* sense of safety and security in their lives. This is why racism in all of its forms in the lives of Black clients has to be a part of a clinician's knowledge base.

Trauma and racism are inextricably linked based on a broad overview of the literature on the role race plays in how people view themselves, the world, and others. There is not a single area of society in American life that has not been impacted by the legacy of racism. Whether it is laws that prohibited where pools could be built to prohibit Blacks from swimming, voting procedures that were designed to increase barriers for Blacks to vote, prohibitions on the way American history is taught, or where one is allowed to live—the impact of slavery, racism, and segregation in America has permeated the experience of our lives to the point that we may not even notice it.

Or, not *all* of us notice it.

Moreover, the impact of racism has been identified by the American Academy of Pediatrics as a social determinant of health, indicating that racism results in youth exposure to stressors and systemic barriers that affect not only their access to care, but also their biology and predisposition to ailments later in life that are tied to inflammation (Trent et al., 2019). **Race-based traumatic stress** can be both direct and indirect. Direct exposure may be interpersonal, such as when a person is called a racial slur, whereas indirect exposure can take the form of **vicarious**

trauma, akin to what Sean experienced when he viewed the video of George Floyd's murder. Though he did not experience the violence himself, he clearly had watched videos like that enough times that they caused him to have understandable panic when he was later pulled over by the police officer.

Key Terms for the Reader

In this book, we discuss the impact of racism and how systemic racism has and can lead to the experience of microaggressions, discrimination, and race-based trauma and traumatic stress. We define these terms here for reference throughout this text. For more on terminology, please see the glossary at the end of the book.

> **Racism:** The 2024 edition of the *Merriam-Webster Dictionary* defines racism as "the systemic oppression of a racial group to the social, economic, and political advantage of another."
> **Microaggressions:** *Merriam-Webster* also defines microaggressions as "a comment or action that subtly and often unconsciously or unintentionally expresses a prejudiced attitude toward a member of a marginalized group (such as a racial minority)."
> **Racial trauma/race-based traumatic stress:** Racial trauma refers to the elevated stress that people of color experience—often unknown to them—that exacerbates symptoms that may have already existed, or newly form, as a result of repeated adverse experiences, related to their race. This includes personal experiences of racism or racial **discrimination**, but has also been linked to vicarious traumatization when witnessing or repeatedly learning of negative racial experiences of people within the same group. For Black clients, seeing the sometimes fatal outcomes of other Black people impacted by racism and discrimination amplifies their fear.

It is critical that as clinicians, we adopt person-centered language when talking about racial trauma in clinical settings. For example, psychologists have been encouraged to shift language and use phrases like "person *with* depression" or "person *affected by trauma*," rather than "depressed person" or "traumatized person." The reason for this was to ensure that a patient's identity is not their illness or experience. To that end, it is important for clinicians to understand that racial trauma is something that *happens to* people. It would not be person-centered language to say that a person or group of people are racially traumatized, but rather that they are affected by race-based traumatic stress. By using this language and understanding that racial trauma, like any other trauma, happens to people, we take the stance as the clinician to help clients understand the systems that have impacted their lives, rather than making their experiences their identities. To do that, we must self-examine and ask ourselves if we actually *believe* racism is something that exists and affects the lives of Black people in America. If you are reading this book, you must have some level of willingness to learn more.

People Are Not Broken, but Systems Are

Gara et al. (2019) published findings from an archival data review of medical records in a large behavioral health care system. Gara concluded that Black patients diagnosed with schizophrenia met criteria for major depression at higher rates than non-Latino whites. Gara went on to hypothesize that routine screening for major depression in community mental health settings may reduce racial disparities in the diagnosing of more severe mental health diagnoses like schizophrenia in Black clients. Barnes (2008) also discussed this phenomenon of Black clients disproportionately being diagnosed and medicated for serious mental illness such as schizophrenia or psychosis when severe depression or other mood disorder may have been a more precise and accurate diagnosis. Gara's work, as well as Barnes's, are consistent with findings from other studies that identified the significant trend of diagnosing Black clients with more severe mental health diagnoses and of underdiagnosing illnesses such as depression, posttraumatic stress disorder (PTSD), obsessive–compulsive disorder (OCD), and the like. What is also so concerning about these findings is that serious mental illnesses like schizophrenia are usually "rule-out" diagnoses, meaning that in order to diagnose them, the symptoms cannot be better accounted for by other mood disorders.

The trend in our field to underdiagnose mood disorders in Black clients specifically means that there is clear bias in how symptom presentation is interpreted by providers. These biases have significant impact: A schizophrenia diagnosis versus one of severe depression is represented very differently to the public and can lead to more **stigmatization** and discrimination. And at a base level, assigning an incorrect diagnosis also means a person would not receive the proper treatment for their presenting problem. In an epidemiological study published in the *American Journal of Public Health*, Gibbs et al. (2013) found that African Americans exhibited more chronic, persistent symptoms of anxiety while also having lower treatment rates and poorer treatment outcomes. Through their research, Gibbs et al. (2013) explained how misdiagnosis stemming from racism leads to cultural mistrust, which could possibly account for decreased likelihood for African Americans to seek treatment. As clinicians, if we are truly committed to doing the nuanced work of recognizing the operation of race-based bias in our field, we must consider this history of misdiagnosis when working with Black clients and examining their mental health histories.

Trends of attributing more severe characteristics to Black people span other sectors of American life beyond mental health. Black children in school settings receive detentions and out- of-school suspensions at higher rates than their white counterparts. (Young & Butler, 2018). As recently as 2016, medical students were found to endorse beliefs about Black patients having higher tolerance for pain, which has resulted in denying these patients pain medication when presenting to hospitals (Hoffman, Trawalter, Axt, & Oliver, 2016; Washington, 2006). The lack of trust in the reporting of symptoms can result in Black patients feeling suspicious of medical health services. In mental health settings, there is evidence of more serious diagnoses being assigned to Black Americans, resulting in their being prescribed stronger medications or more frequently being referred for hospitalization than white patients with similar symptom profiles. Biases about Black people in mental health settings also result in their being labeled as "difficult" or "noncompliant," based on their behavior and decisions stemming from their mistrust of health care systems. Similarly, Black youth are more likely to be labeled as "oppositional" or "psychotic" than their white counterparts (Gara et al., 2019; Washington, 2006; Henderson et al., 2015).

Clinicians working with Black clients should consider the impact of bias by reflecting on our own training. How much formal training did we get in our graduate programs about race-based traumatic stress? Although the terms "complex trauma" and "trauma-informed care" are common in mental health care agencies, many education programs in behavioral health devote a handful of lectures, if that many, to discussion specifically about trauma—for the general population. Discussions about race are often relegated to an end-of-semester lecture, treated as a special topic of sorts. With the gaps in culturally focused training for students in clinical training programs, practitioners have to seek additional knowledge and experience to understand the impact of bias, discrimination, and systemic racism in other ways—frequently, postgraduate studies and jobs. Clinicians looking for more training on race-based trauma can find it by seeking literature and continuing education opportunities that are specific to the topic. The clinicians who seek these training and experiential opportunities are self-selecting, of course, already recognizing how important and valuable these topics and considerations are to their work as clinicians.

Clinicians and graduate students in training can also engage in experiential learning in both formal and informal settings. Comfort with talking about unfamiliar or uncomfortable topics is necessary for mental health providers, and conversations about race should be viewed no differently. The more practice one engages in, the better one becomes. The topics outlined in this text can offer some ideas on how to take advantage of clinical opportunities to talk about race, racism, discrimination, and the like with clients.

Looking at Your Own Racial Identity

As Kenneth Hardy clarifies: "Our difficulty [in meeting the needs of youth of color in treatment] is not just because of greater 'pathology' or 'resistance' as some assert. Rather, we fail to appreciate the ways in which race is entangled in their suffering" (Hardy, 2013, p. 24). When Hardy (2023) explains this concept, he refers to it as "invisible wounds." These wounds may not even be understood by those scarred by them, for lots of reasons we will discuss in this and subsequent chapters. Clinicians who understand these wounds will better conceptualize the client's reported experience while considering the backdrop of racism and its sometimes blatant—but often insidious—role in a client's clinical presentation.

In the book *Racial Trauma: Clinical Strategies and Techniques for Healing Invisible Wounds* (2023), Hardy discusses seven invisible wounds of racial trauma. They are internalized devaluation, an assaulted sense of self, psychological homelessness, voicelessness, loss and collective grief, orientation toward survival, and rage. Hardy also emphasizes that in order for clinicians to be able to address racial trauma, they must first engage in self-reflection and adopt a racial lens. This makes sense because if a clinician understands their own **racial identity** and the areas of power and **privilege** in the spaces they occupy, they can more comfortably have conversations about these topics. Our role as clinicians, after all, is to be able to have the tough conversations that the friends, family, or acquaintances of our clients may not want or be able to have. If we shy away from the topic, clients may sense our hesitation, making the therapy room yet another unsafe space for them. In Sean's case, one of his self-reported symptoms was the need to be perfect. People who are perfectionists are often good at sensing if they are approved or disapproved by someone. If he senses a clinician's unwillingness to address trauma, racism, or discrimination, he may not bring it up in an effort to spare the clinician from having to bring up the topic, which only worsens the wound of having to appear perfect and pulled together, even when he is scared and anxious.

Using a Racial Trauma Lens to Conceptualize Sean's Case

It is likely that Sean could go to a therapist for treatment about his anxiety and the subject of his race never comes up. From psychotherapy research, we know that clinicians will often not ask clients about things they are not familiar with or feel incapable of treating. Because Sean is coming into treatment years after he was pulled over by a policeman and had an intense feeling of fear, he may not even realize how the traffic stop affected him. And if history has taught us anything, it is likely that he has continued to experience or bear witness to racial injustices during the time that has elapsed since that encounter with police as a teenager.

There are myriad direct and indirect ways that a clinician could approach Sean therapeutically that will facilitate discussion about his experiences related to race, racism, and discrimination. These talks can then connect to his presenting issue of anxiety. For clinicians that are just beginning to focus on integrating these conversations in their therapeutic style, it may feel more comfortable to be less direct and to give space for Sean to bring questions about race and racism to the forefront. Skilled clinicians with more experience and comfort having targeted discussions about race may take a more direct approach. Either approach can be fruitful. And if nothing else, either sends a message to the client that the clinician is willing and able to talk about what many in the public domain deem to be taboo or too provocative to discuss outside of family and friend circles. Here are some ways that a clinician can ask a client about the impact of race and culture:

INDIRECT PROMPTS

"Can you tell me more about prior times in your life where you felt very anxious or fearful?"

"Tell me more about your family. What were some of the important lessons/values you grew up with?"

"You mentioned you feel like you have to be perfect at work and you don't trust your coworkers. Can you say more about that? What is the risk of making mistakes?"

DIRECT PROMPTS

"In what ways has your identity or cultural background impacted your expectations of yourself?" (Identities can include sex, gender, race, religion, etc.)

"I know that in many Black families, children learn about how to be in spaces where they may encounter prejudice or race-related stress. Was this your experience?" (If affirmative, inquire about how that has affected the client's life in positive and challenging ways.)

These are just a few examples; we'll present more later in the book. By broaching topics of race and culture early on in treatment, at least making it known to a client like Sean that the clinician is comfortable talking about these topics, the therapist can help him to feel like the therapy room is a place where he can have more control and comfort in what is discussed. Trauma—in all of its forms—results in a person feeling an overwhelming loss of control, predictability, power over self, and psychological safety (Blaustein & Kinniburgh, 2018). Incorporating elements into therapy sessions like control, comfort, and ability to set the pace of the interaction can help healing begin.

Thinking Ahead: Approaches to Care

Understanding race-based traumatic stress can help us to think more creatively about how to apply treatment approaches in more culturally responsive ways. It could be easy for a clinician who uses a more cognitive-behavioral approach to aim to help Sean identify his cognitive distortions and to challenge automatic thoughts. But should he challenge them? What is at risk if he does that? Are such cognitions distorted? Or, is Sean's need to be "perfect" and steer clear of work colleagues a strategy for survival that has worked well for him, even though the result is severe anxiety and social isolation? As noted earlier, part of your therapeutic approach may be to let the client lead and share what is on their mind with infrequent interruption from you in a session. Would Sean treat that as an opportunity to show that he is a "good patient"? Would he come in each week with an agenda of his talking points and seek your reassurance that he is doing therapy the *right* way? In the next chapter, we will talk about how interventions can be updated and adapted to better meet the needs of Black clients.

In this chapter, we discussed the foundational knowledge that helps us, as providers, to understand the undercurrent of racism that can impact the worldview and coping strategies employed by Black clients. Again, understanding this information is not meant to engage in reductionist approaches to mental health care. As with any approach to treatment, tailoring to the individual experiences of Black clients is important. In subsequent chapters, we discuss how clinicians can improve their skills in identifying whether and how racism, discrimination, racial trauma, and microaggressions impact the lives of Black clients in therapy.

CHAPTER TAKEAWAYS

- Trauma and racism are inextricably linked, as racism permeates so many facets of American life. For Black clients, while they may not readily identify racism or race-based stress as central to their presenting problem, a clinician can consider it in conceptualizing their case if they have reason to believe that it will help them better understand their client's experience.

- Racial trauma is *not* a diagnosis. Rather, racial trauma can impact the severity of diagnosable mental health conditions, and conceptualizing a case using a racial trauma lens may aid the clinician in taking approaches to care that are culturally responsive.

- While clinicians may have concerns about broaching subjects such as race and other cultural factors impacting their clients, raising such topics may help to promote more connection between them and clients who are experiencing distress that might be linked to racism, discrimination, or microaggressions.

CHAPTER 2

Thinking Outside the Box
Treatment Adaptations to Address Racial Trauma

> Because we do not know how to talk to strangers,
> what do we do when things go awry with strangers?
> We blame the stranger.
> —MALCOLM GLADWELL (2019)

Think back to your foundational coursework in your graduate psychology training programs. Remember active and reflective listening, Socratic questioning, engagement, and rapport building? For those trained to be mental health practitioners, the message was that these necessary skills were key to establishing a connection with clients and achieving that critical therapeutic alliance that lends itself to positive outcomes for our clients. Essentially, we learned how to talk to strangers. You may also recall discussions about "resistant," "noncompliant," or "treatment-resistant" clients, as well as "transference" and "countertransference." But how many of us discussed **implicit** and **explicit bias**? What about the impact of racism and discrimination in our practice of mental health treatment was included in our coursework? And if so, was it discussed in the context of the application of evidence-based treatment models and their implementation? For many courses of study in the area of behavioral health disciplines, up until recent years, the concept of culture was often relegated to the final lectures at the end of a semester, as opposed to a concept threaded throughout the course. In the past several years, the stigma of seeking treatment for mental health issues has steadily lessened, with more diverse populations seeking therapy. For Black clients, the reasons for seeking treatment are generally similar to the reasons people from other populations seek treatment: struggles with anxiety, depression, work/school stress, addictive behaviors, relationship distress, and so forth. An added layer for Black clients, however, is the impact of discrimination and racism in their everyday lives, an impact that makes those stressors feel inescapable.

Racism and discrimination are systemic issues that are not dismantled by just one clinician working with a client. Even with a little understanding of how these issues operate, it may feel daunting for the therapist to consider how to address them. And yet, it *is* possible to consider and integrate the impact of racism into widely used therapeutic approaches. We would argue that it is not only possible, but also crucial to effective therapy practice. As a start, clinicians need to consider where they can grow their knowledge in the areas of cultural competence and cultural humility.

Cultural Competence and Cultural Humility

Cultural competence has been defined as behaviors, attitudes, and policies that, when taken together, work to ensure that systems and people within those systems can engage with diverse cultural groups appropriately and in an efficient manner. This definition by the U.S. Department of Health and Human Services (HSS) Health Resources and Services Administration (HRSA) was included in Green-Moten and Minkler's article (2020) about the debate between the terms "cultural competence" and "cultural humility." Cultural humility is a concept initially attributed to the writings of Tervalon and Murray-Garcia (1998). **Cultural humility** is less about increasing competence in understanding the culture of others, but rather emphasizes the commitment a person makes to engage in self-reflection and recognize power imbalances that exist and they participate in to ensure improved and equitable experiences on behalf of others who do not benefit from these power dynamics (Tervalon & Murray-Garcia, 1998).

While the literature sometimes discusses the concepts of cultural competence and humility as qualitatively different skill sets, for clinicians interested in ensuring that issues concerning race and racism are integrated into treatments, both concepts—interwoven together—can add much value to the quality of care for Black clients. Clinicians who are self-reflective, recognize the impact of power and privilege that they and others hold, and have worked to increase their competence in discussing diversity and issues related to race and culture will likely approach—rather than avoid—conversations with their Black clients about their exposure to racism, discrimination, and stereotypes in their everyday lives. In this chapter, we discuss ways to do this.

Historical Context

The history of psychological treatment approaches is overwhelmingly Eurocentric and patriarchal in nature. In the classic work *Even the Rat Was White: A Historical View of Psychology* (Guthrie, 2004), the timeline of psychological research and treatment implementation is examined, highlighting the shortcomings of the field of psychology in respecting and including Black people. The impact of this is still felt in the field today, with many widely used treatment models initially developed in research studies that were not inclusive of representative populations, Black people in particular. The lack of representation of Black research participants in psychological studies is due to many factors. Some aspects are systemic in nature and others are related to personal choice. From a systemic perspective, much of the early-20th-century psychological treatment and theory research took place in a university setting, a place where many Black people were not even permitted to be because of segregation laws. Furthermore, early research did not include Black subjects, and this can be attributed to the failure to recognize Black people as *people*; thus, their exclusion from research is notable, as outlined in Guthrie's work.

Many efficacy studies for some of the most widely used treatments for the most commonly diagnosed psychiatric illnesses were originally designed with samples that excluded more than the most complex of comorbid disorders. People from communities of color were also not a part of these early studies. Clinical treatments have a history of being created for and by people who represent the majority culture, and in the case of the United States, that means white and cisgender male populations (Sue, 1999). As a result, the experiences of historically marginalized groups are underrepresented in the development of these treatments, diagnoses, and can negatively impact treatment outcomes for Black people. This is not to say that these treatments do not work with Black clients; as we know through study repetition and effectiveness studies, these treatments can be widely effective with diverse populations. But when treatments do NOT work, what do we do? This chapter will explore the most prominent examples of diagnostic and treatment trends that result in poor outcomes or reduced treatment-seeking behaviors for Black people, and how clinicians can adapt treatment to better serve Black clients and discuss the impact of race and culture on their mental health.

Before the Intervention Is Self-Reflection

Calloway and Creed (2022) call for a shift in how culturally responsive care is viewed in the field in terms of service delivery, especially in light of the increased engagement of communities of color with the behavioral health sector. The authors highlight that the field must shift to no longer designating culturally responsive learning as an elective option for those entering the field, but rather a core competency that is required and threaded into all courses of study. In the example below, we feature a few of these strategies for such integration in commonly used therapeutic interventions. First, let's explore how therapists can increase their competency by broaching the subject of culture with Black clients. One approach, **reflective local practice (RLP)**, helps a provider to engage in self-reflection to better understand themselves so they can be more intentional and mindful when discussing cultural identity issues with clients.

Sandeen et al. (2018) developed the concept of RLP as an answer to the need to have a pragmatic way of teaching cultural competence for trainees in the field of mental health. It was considered a strategy that could be helpful for clients and for trainees. Essentially, the title of the approach is a directive. Psychologists and training programs that adopt this approach should primarily focus on being reflective, engaging in self-study of their own cultural identities and how that impacts their practices and beliefs. Next, there should be an understanding of the *local culture* that practitioners and training programs are serving. Included in this understanding should be awareness of the historical contexts that contribute to the current local culture. And finally, the last component is *practice* in talking about culture with clients. This includes role plays in practicing broaching the subject of culture with clients, learning how to discuss racism with clients, and how to handle a situation when a rupture occurs as a result of cultural differences with a client.

This approach is a primer for the cultural adaptations and implementations of psychological interventions because it helps therapists to be able to start the process by first discussing cultural identity and differences. (For more on RLP, see Chapter 4.) As we noted, Black clients are more likely to encounter racism and discrimination, which impacts their mental health. So when a Black individual comes to a mental health provider, they should not consider the therapist's cultural competence or responsiveness to be a "specialty," but rather, an expected part of their treatment, a provider who can openly and comfortably discuss race and discrimination. Sometimes this very discussion is about the racial difference between the provider and the client, and other times, it may be the need to talk about the impact of everyday discrimination on the life of the client. Whatever the issue, for Black clients, the therapeutic alliance may be on the line if the therapist is either ignoring discussion of race and discrimination altogether, or worse, waiting for the client to bring it up themself.

For example, if a Black client in treatment is presenting with issues about work stress and balancing their personal life with work, a therapist who is attuned to the impact of race and discrimination may integrate questions about these issues and how they may impact work.

> THERAPIST: You mentioned that your job is really stressful. Can you share a little more about that?
>
> CLIENT: Yes, I am a project manager and it seems like we keep having large jobs to execute back to back without much reprieve, and I feel like there is a lot on me to constantly produce without having a breather. Everyone expects a lot from me, from my team to my supervisor.

THERAPIST: That does sound like it can be overwhelming, and I could see how that can play into your challenges with trying to balance work and your personal life. Can you tell me a little bit more about your job and who you work with?

CLIENT: Yes, I am the lead for my team, and I have about four people who report to me.

THERAPIST: In some work settings that are high-pressure like what you are describing, there can also be personality differences that make work that much more challenging. Is that your experience? Do you feel like your team is cohesive and that you are respected as a leader?

CLIENT: Sometimes. I am actually the youngest person on my team, so sometimes that gets in the way. I am also the only Black male, only Black person. So I am constantly feeling like I am under a microscope because of my age and race. I worked really hard to get where I am and want to do well.

THERAPIST: Tell me a bit more about that experience if you think that would help me understand more about your current stress. . . .

The therapist's ability to use what the client shares to further understand the presenting problem shows the client that all the information they share is relevant to the therapist understanding them as a whole person. That connection in the early stages of treatment and genuine openness to learning are the building blocks for a strong therapeutic alliance.

Adaptations of Treatment Approaches That Address Race-Based Traumatic Stress

The approaches below have evidence-based results for positive effects on treating trauma in youth and adults. Clinicians who are utilizing these interventions can integrate discussion and assessment of the impact of race and racism in the lives of Black clients.

Trauma-Focused Cognitive-Behavioral Therapy

As a gold standard treatment for youth who have experienced traumatic events, trauma-focused cognitive-behavioral therapy (TF-CBT) is widely used in the field of behavioral health and has been found to be effective with many different populations. Metzger et al. (2021) described strategies to map onto the TF-CBT treatment components to factor in racial socialization for African American clients. Racial socialization is the intergenerational process of transmitting messages to children about African American culture, attitudes, and belief systems as it relates to how to survive in a world that holds deeply entrenched racism and discrimination toward them. It is a method of preparing youth to cope with these inevitable stressors in an effort to protect them. Metzger and her colleagues suggest exploring the client's and family's beliefs related to their racial identity and delving into culturally relevant strategies, such as relaxation practices, for example. Another way of adapting this treatment to include the impact of racial identity is in the treatment component focused on affective expression; clinicians can give space for clients to discuss their emotions when they have encountered racial discrimination.

One treatment component of TF-CBT is psychoeducation about trauma for both the youth and the caregiver. In the example below, the clinician integrates aspects of racism and discrimination into this education, with the intention of giving space for involved family members to be comfortable talking about racial and cultural issues if and when needed:

> THERAPIST: As you know, today we will be talking about some basic facts about trauma and issues related to trauma so that we can rely on that knowledge as we move forward in the treatment process. This discussion today will also help you to see that the traumatic experiences you have lived through have happened to others—so much so that we have data and school curriculum about it. You are definitely not alone in your experience, even though it can feel that way. [In this introduction, the therapist is providing context about what is about to happen, which builds safety in the therapeutic interaction. The therapist is also providing validating statements in advance for the

client to reduce the feelings of stigma and shame that are often associated with traumatic stress.]

THERAPIST: *(later in the session)* OK, so I have shared some facts and information about how frequently traumatic events happen to young people and how it affects them. There are sometimes other aspects of our lives that can make our feelings and reactions to these traumatic events even more stressful. Experiencing racism and discrimination can also be a type of stressor that can be just as hard, if not harder, to cope with because it may feel like there is no relief from it. There is a concept called race-based traumatic stress that can affect Black people and other people of color when they are dealing with discrimination or witnessing negative events that affect people that look like them, and these situations can make going through the type of trauma you are coming here for even harder to manage. Examples of small ways that racial trauma can affect you are when people make assumptions about your credibility because of your race, or show less concern for your emotional and physical pain. You may feel like you or your parent have to plead your case to others to get the help you need because people do not have empathy for the pain you are dealing with. Let's talk about how your life is impacted by your cultural background. Tell me a little bit about whether or not you feel you have been impacted by these issues. . . .

In this example, the therapist is aiming to help the client see how race and the experience of racism can show up in subtle ways, thereby educating the client and caregiver and demonstrating the therapist's own comfort with broaching the subject. For many Black clients, and with the ubiquitous nature of systemic racism, a therapist should not assume that Black clients are so obviously aware of how these systems affect their lives. By bringing it up in treatment, the therapist is providing the psychoeducation and may be offering the client and caregiver a chance to look at their posttraumatic stress in a different light, willing to explore how racism and discrimination exacerbate symptoms of trauma.

Overall, for a youth-focused treatment like TF-CBT, adapting the treatment components to explore the impact of racial identity and encounters with discrimination and bias *adds value* to the treatment experience for the family. Metzger further describes topic areas that may be clinically indicated to assess and build interventions for, such as experiences of sexualization and adultification of young Black girls that are often an important factor when sexual abuse occurs, intersectionality issues (e.g., being Black and gay, Black and a woman), or the impact of microaggressions and racist beliefs within multiracial families and their extended relatives.

Cognitive-Behavioral Therapy

In the behavioral health field, cognitive-behavioral therapy (CBT) is another widely used approach shown to be effective in the treatment of a variety of presenting issues like depression, anxiety, and so on. Core concepts in the CBT approach include psychoeducation about the presenting concerns, exploration of automatic thoughts, core beliefs, and coping strategies, among other concepts (Beck & Wright, 1997). The clinician's role in CBT is to be a guide in a coaching role, metaphorically, to help the client explore the validity of dysfunctional beliefs about themself, the world, and others. Cultural adaptations of CBT have been found to be helpful for African American clients in several ways (Steele & Newton, 2022). For example, some Black clients presenting in treatment may have anxious thoughts that are rooted in internalized messages, in turn, rooted in racism. Thoughts about being effective in their jobs or school, fears about being their authentic selves with others without judgment, or thoughts of not fitting in or being good enough are examples of these types of internalized feelings. Strategies the clinician might consider broaching are automatic thoughts and core beliefs being a function of internalized messages that are rooted in a client's racial identity. In the following example, the client is a 40-year-old African American woman experiencing stress at work and trying to balance her work and social life.

> THERAPIST: You recently shared that one of your biggest stressors right now is trying to balance your work and your social life. Can you say more about that?

CLIENT: Yes, my job is very demanding and sometimes requires me to work weird hours because some of our partners are based in other time zones both within and outside of the United States. I feel like I always have to be "on" and accessible at all times. If not, it will look like I am slacking off and I can't have that perception of me out there. I worked too hard to get to my current position to be in that situation.

THERAPIST: When you say you have to be "on" or it will look like you are slacking off, is that what YOU would think about yourself, or are you saying that is what others will think?

CLIENT: Maybe both? I know I definitely would be worried others would think that, but maybe I would think it, too.

THERAPIST: When you say that you have to be "on," or will be perceived this way, where does that thought come from?

CLIENT: I think it comes from just knowing I am one of the only Black managers there AND I am a woman in a male-dominated world. While no one has ever directly said anything to make me feel that way, the fact that there are hardly any Black people in leadership makes me feel like I have to step it up, have to be on point and better than good.

THERAPIST: Where did you learn that this is how you need to be?

CLIENT: Just through osmosis, I guess! (*laughs*) No, but I think as a kid growing up, my parents really tried to help me understand everything the people before me and them went through so I could have the opportunities I have and not to take things for granted. They taught me that I need to work even harder and put in 110%, not 100%. It wasn't like pressure or anything like that. It was more like I needed to be grateful and my success showed that gratitude and respect.

THERAPIST: That is actually a really great perspective to have. When you say where it comes from, it seems like it comes from a very positive space. And then at the same time, when you talk about how that translates into how you talk to yourself and about work expectations, it turns into something that sounds more overwhelming. Is that right?

CLIENT: Yes, maybe. I think as time went on, I began to think that if I am not successful and the best and not always on top of things, I was letting people down. Even letting myself down. I need to do the absolute most and then every time I do well and reach another success, it's like "OK, how do I top that?" It's just a constant need to be top-tier, always. It has definitely spiraled into something else.

THERAPIST: It sounds exhausting. But it also sounds like it is actually coming from a place of honoring those who did so much so you could have the opportunity. I am wondering if there is room to hold both that gratitude and also give yourself the opportunity to breathe and enjoy what they worked so hard for you to do. Is it your interpretation that showing gratitude meant you could not rest?

CLIENT: I don't know. I never thought about it. I think if I don't give that 110% every time, that I will mess up my progress or be seen as not working hard enough. I don't want to give any of my colleagues ammunition to say that I am being lazy or standoffish or anything. Taking a day off or even leaving email and things alone when I am not at work does not feel like an option.

THERAPIST: Because if you take those breaks or lean back a bit from work, what will happen?

CLIENT: I will miss something important and then my job can be at risk?

THERAPIST: Is that a definite outcome? You said you *will*.

CLIENT: Well, it *may*. That is probably more likely.

THERAPIST: Can I ask how many times when you have, for example, checked your email all weekend, has there been something major that you would have missed had you not checked it?

CLIENT: Not many times. Actually, hardly ever. And if there was, someone would have probably texted me if it was major.

THERAPIST: So then, what does saying that out loud feel like when you reflect on this need to be "on" all the time?

CLIENT: I think this is an example where things are in my head about what I need to do, but I may not actually need to do those things to still be seen as "on." It's not like I am missing things or flaking out on the job.

In this example, the therapist is engaging in some cognitive restructuring: examining evidence for or against the automatic thoughts related to how this client views their productivity and drive in their work life. By helping the client to explore where the source of these thoughts may be coming from, the client is able to see the paradox of her wanting and needing to show gratitude and respect for ancestors who fought for her to experience the opportunities she currently has, but she is not allowing herself to enjoy her successes and make time for herself to enjoy the fruits of her labor. If the clinician wanted to go further to deepen the cultural component, they may try to circle back to the unhelpful thoughts and have the client engage in more exploration of the source of her drive:

THERAPIST: When you think about your ancestors and what they fought for so you and those before you could have opportunities, do you think they would be disappointed in you taking time off or enjoying a break? Would it feel like you wasted their efforts?

CLIENT: I mean, I guess they might feel like it's a luxury because Lord knows, they were not able to take breaks when they were enslaved. And even their descendants—they were working the fields and tough labor jobs where if they didn't go to work, they didn't make the pennies they were paid. The things they did led to my generation having jobs that give us time off and whatnot. I haven't ever really thought that far to ask myself, "Well, would my ancestors think I am lazy or wasting opportunity?" It sounds a little wild as I am breaking this down right now.

THERAPIST: This is a helpful exercise whenever you start to feel anxious or pressure to perform. Checking in with yourself about what you are telling yourself and then asking about the veracity of those thoughts or where the source of them lies may help you to put things in perspective.

For clinicians familiar with cognitive-behavioral therapy, one could paraphrase that an aim of the treatment is to identify and dispel persisting cognitions that result in overestimation of threat paired with a feeling of inability to cope. Some of the typical CBT language is not used in the above example intentionally. Some African American clients may have automatic thoughts with themes related to fears of behaving in ways that may affirm stereotypes (e.g., being perceived as lazy or aggressive) but are not necessarily irrational. Rather, these are fear-based thoughts rooted in very real messages and biases that have existed for generations about Black Americans, even though they are unfounded stereotypes. For a Black woman who is a professional in a corporate environment, it is not beyond the realm of reason that she may hold added layers of worry about how her actions will be perceived by colleagues who are not Black (and even by those who are not women). So, a typical CBT intervention (e.g., cognitive restructuring) to assess evidence for and against that worry—in the absence of considering her identities of race and gender and the realities of bias in the workplace—would be an oversight on the part of the therapist. Instead of taking the usual CBT approach, it may be more helpful to focus more on what the client's internal dialogue is and where those messages are coming from in the first place. This can help lead the clinician to focus on core beliefs held by the client and also helps the clinician understand the impact of racial messages and fears about bias in the life of the client. If the therapist took the route of having the client explore what her coworkers have said or done, it could appear as if the therapist is coming to the rescue of her coworkers or being an apologist for them if they are, in fact, putting pressure on the client to perform at a higher expectation than they have for themselves.

Integration of Techniques from Differing Orientations

Scharff et al. (2021) found that in addition to Black clients' preference for Black therapists, Black therapists also report better therapeutic outcomes for their clients if they integrate cognitive-behavioral strategies with psychodynamic/interpersonal interventions, such as integration of social justice issues and their impact on the life of the client, incorporation of spirituality, and constantly focusing on the building and maintenance of the therapeutic alliance. Incorporating CBT strategies can be helpful because for many Black clients, the concrete skills and interventions offered by CBT help to understand and problem-solve issues related to anxiety, mood challenges, and other problems. In tandem with psychodynamic/interpersonal interventions, this integration of approaches can help to strengthen the client's connection to the therapist. The relationship and exploration of the client's personal history help the therapeutic alliance, which leads to optimal outcomes. Clinicians must be open to this type of integration in order better connect with clients.

Revisiting the example of the woman coping with issues at work, the client broached the subject of race *before* the therapist did. In the following example, the therapist instead approaches the subject first and explores the impact of race in the client's perceptions of herself and may believe others have on her.

> THERAPIST: You mentioned that you feel like you always have to be "on" at work? What does that mean to you?
>
> CLIENT: That I have to be on top of all of my work, never falling behind, and maintaining my emotions while there. Like, even if someone makes a mistake that impacts me or creates more work for me, I have to overthink how I react.
>
> THERAPIST: That does sound really stressful. You had mentioned that you are a manager. Are there other managers who share your same level of stress? I know sometimes beyond just the role, other aspects of our identities can impact how others perceive us and even how we perceive ourselves.

In this moment, the therapist is moving toward opening a discussion about identities that could include the client's race and gender. It also gives the client the option *not* to discuss it.

> CLIENT: I think my stress at work, in part, comes from just knowing I am one of the only Black managers there AND I am a woman

in a male-dominated world. While no one has ever directly said anything to make me feel that way, the fact that there are hardly any Black people in leadership makes me feel like I have to step it up, have to be on point and better than good.

THERAPIST: First, I want to thank you for mentioning that because your explanation really helps me understand how your race and gender identity, taken together, affect how you feel when you are at work. What I heard you say there is that even though no one has directly said anything about you being Black and a woman in your position, you recognize that those aspects of who you are impact the way you function in the workplace. Is that accurate?

CLIENT: Yes, absolutely.

In this exchange, the use of the client's words and reflecting back what was heard is an example of the kinds of basic interpersonal skills that clinicians use as a method to foster a therapeutic alliance and help the client feel heard and understood.

Throughout this book, clinicians will learn strategies for adapting treatment and offering consultation to individuals, families, and communities to support Black clients and communities looking to mitigate the impact of racism and discrimination on Black people.

CHAPTER TAKEAWAYS

- Training programs in behavioral health fall short in preparing therapists to feel competent in discussing culture and identity with clients. For Black clients, this can potentially result in a weak therapeutic alliance, as the therapist may not be willing or even able to discuss the impact of everyday discrimination and racism that add layers to mental health challenges. Cultural competence and humility should not be elective options in training programs any longer.

- Approaches like reflective local practice (RLP) provide therapists with the skills to increase comfort in talking about culture and help them recognize where they have biases when it comes to working with Black clients.

- Integration of race and culture discussions can help optimize the therapeutic experience for Black clients. Having space in therapy to talk about how race and messages about race impact their thoughts, emotions, and behaviors helps these clients feel validation and builds a sense of trust and willingness to try suggested interventions.

CHAPTER 3

Awareness in Action
Understanding the Barriers and Facilitators to Treatment Seeking

> It is not uncommon for the oppressed to suffer in silence with considerable degrees of underlying angst, humiliation, despair, depression, and rage—all without appropriate channels for expression and discharge.
> —Ken Hardy (2023)

Mark and Jessica Smith are seeking treatment to help their 14-year-old daughter, Alexis, deal with stress related to school and social interactions. Alexis has reportedly been struggling with perfectionism at school, taking longer than necessary to complete assignments, and is "obsessed" with going to a top-tier college, even though she is only in the middle of her freshman year of high school. Mark and Jessica also have two other children, Chris (age 20, currently in college), and Erica (age 12, who is in the 7th grade). Alexis avoids peer interactions because, although she wants to feel like she is a part of a nice group of friends, they often say and do things that remind her that she is the only Black girl in the group. They make comments about her hair, how she talks, or they talk in ways that make her feel like they are mocking her culture. She attends school and lives in a predominantly white school district, and her parents believe that is part of why she struggles with her sense of belonging. In addition to this, Mark and Jessica have struggled to identify strategies to help their two daughters navigate some of the challenges of the school and the academically rigorous environment, which exacerbates Alexis's anxiety related to her schoolwork. Alexis presents as a friendly, talkative child. She enumerates all her accomplishments and hobbies during the first meeting and, when asked why she thinks her parents have brought her to therapy, she shrugs and mentions that they think she is too anxious. Mark and Jessica mentioned that they have considered therapy for Alexis for at least 3 years but were hesitant for lots of reasons.

Why was the Smith family reluctant to seek therapy when they noticed their daughter Alexis's challenges a couple of years ago? What would a therapist explore with them in terms of parenting their child? How would a therapist talk with Alexis about the current challenges she faces, and what are the underlying reasons for these challenges? This chapter will focus on the individual and systems-level barriers that Black clients experience when seeking treatment for mental health challenges and how racial trauma factors into those barriers. Additionally, there is discussion about changes that individual clinicians and psychological treatment organizations can make to reduce barriers and increase engagement with Black clients.

The process of finding a therapist has always proven challenging for anyone, regardless of race. According to research, one of the key factors in successful therapy is not the type of clinical orientation or evidence-based practice that the clinician uses. Rather, the *fit* between clinician and client is identified as being one of the most important predictors of client outcomes. The relationship—what we call the "therapeutic alliance"—is significant (Baier, Kline, & Feeny, 2020). But for a relationship to begin, a client and clinician must find each other.

For Black clients, some of the barriers to finding a clinician have multiple roots. Joy DeGruy-Leary wrote about the preeminent role that relationships play for the success of African Americans. In her words, "Relationship trumps everything else" (DeGruy-Leary, 2017). In DeGruy's preeminent work *Post Traumatic Slave Syndrome* (2017), she highlights the historical context and socialization of African American culture's high value for kinship and extended families as a protective factor for preserving our sense of self and security. We will discuss more about these historical concepts throughout this book, but the point helps us to understand the importance of the alliance, or lack thereof, in the potential entry into, and maintenance of, mental health treatment for Black clients.

Black clients have been found to be less likely to seek treatment for mental health conditions in outpatient settings but are more likely to seek emergency services for them. Black clients are also more likely to terminate treatment before a mutually agreed upon time with their therapist. Why is this the case? Some of the reasons relate to the existence of more barriers to treatment than facilitators (Ayalon & Alvidrez, 2009). Considering that only 5% of psychologists are Black, according to the American Psychological Association (APA, 2022), most Black clients seeking the help of a psychologist are likely to end up receiving treatment from a white clinician. Black Americans also experience the highest lifetime prevalence of **posttraumatic stress disorder (PTSD)**: at the rate of 8.7%, which is higher than that for every other racial group, including other ethnic minority groups (Roberts, Gilman, Breslau, Breslau, & Kroenen, 2012). This statistic makes sense if we consider what is known about the factors that contribute to prolonged stress symptoms related to trauma. Ford et al. (2006), among other studies, found that prolonged distress and complex symptoms of trauma are higher in prevalence when a trauma exposure is interpersonal in nature. Sometimes, individuals may not necessarily meet the criteria for PTSD, but still struggle with symptoms related to emotional regulation and psychosocial impairment. Although for many mental health clinicians, those who have been studying the impact of racism and discrimination contributing to higher risks for mental health challenges, this is not a new issue, practitioners in the fields of behavioral and medical health have only recently begun citing racism as a major contributor to health outcomes for Black clients.

The concern with this is that in a post-2020 America—where the worst outcomes of the COVID-19 pandemic disproportionately affected Black people, along with the ramifications of the murders of George Floyd, Breonna Taylor, and others, and the political divides in the nation widening—how can clinicians ensure they are aware of the types of issues that may be impacting Black clients who are seeking treatment? In 2022, the U.S. Substance Abuse and Mental Health Services Administration (SAMHSA) published the results of a national survey on substance use and mental health. The data on African Americans indicate a rising increase in depression and serious mental illness, particularly among African American youth (SAMHSA, 2022). How can clinicians work together through their individual networks, state and national psychological associations, and continuing education organizations to ensure that all clinicians are working on culturally responsive treatment when in a cross-racial client–clinician relationship?

Finding a Therapist Who Understands the Impact of Culture on the Experience of Black Clients

One of the barriers potential Black clients encounter is that a clinician may not be able to understand some of their experiences because they do not share their cultural background. While it may be ideal to say that any skilled clinician who understands the importance of therapeutic alliance should be able to treat any client, this is not a realistic perspective. If we, as clinicians, are being honest with ourselves, much of our training is routed in theories and ideals that are Westernized, Eurocentric, and conservative in nature. Theories related to parenting styles, the core ingredients for a healthy relationship, the diagnostic symptomology of conditions like anxiety and depression, and even the widely accepted coping strategies we learn in our training are often from a lens that is generally from the aforementioned cultural perspectives. When potential clients seek a mental health professional, they are usually looking for someone who they ultimately believe will understand them and their problems. For Black clients, particularly in these years since the COVID-19 pandemic and the sociopolitical unrest in the aftermath of George Floyd's murder, the contentious 2020 U.S. presidential election, and insurrection at the U.S. Capitol on January 6, 2021, the experiences of Black clients may represent the psychological fatigue of experiencing a historical onslaught of direct and vicarious traumas. These traumas—rooted in the realities of the disproportionate loss of life in the Black community during the acute stages of the pandemic, and what has been widely accepted as race-based traumatic stress at the heart of other social issues in recent years—only further illustrate this country's long-standing struggle to both avoid and atone for its long history of racial turmoil.

The Stigma of Seeking Treatment for Mental Health Problems

The decision to enter therapy is often hard for anyone, regardless of race. Though the situation is improving, thanks to more celebrities and social media influencers openly talking about therapy and its impact on their quality of life, the decision to seek a mental health professional can still feel like an admission of something being *wrong*. For Black clients, a general theme over the years is that mental health conditions like anxiety and depression are things that can be dealt with either through connection with friends and family, or through guidance from their spiritual faith—not going to a therapist. In the book *Black Families in Therapy* (2013), Nancy Boyd-Franklin highlights some of the barriers for Black clients in seeking mental health services. Among those barriers, she describes suspicion and beliefs about keeping family secrets within the family as being a part of them. Since therapy often involves divulging secrets and letting down one's proverbial guard, it makes sense that the careful selection of therapists is critical for Black clients because, implicitly, the therapist needs to understand that these concerns are entering into the treatment with the client. Or at least if a therapist is using that culturally sensitive lens, they will bring an approach that includes an opportunity to explore these potential concerns at the onset of treatment.

Other barriers that impact Black clients include lack of knowledge about the types of mental health services available and what options exist for them to get help for mental health conditions. This issue can likely be tied to the fact that most people's knowledge of therapy and what it may look like is often tied to whatever images exist in the public that depict therapy. These depictions are usually present in TV shows, films, theater, and literature. As the stigma of seeking therapy has lessened in some communities, clinicians can assume that most clients are not always sure about what their therapy experiences should and could be.

In revisiting the case of Alexis, a therapist may consider this approach during initial conversations with the family:

> THERAPIST: Mark and Jessica, you mentioned that you were hesitant to seek therapy services. Can you say a little bit more about

what your concerns were? [Creates an opportunity for the client to share what barriers may exist without imposing assumptions about why or ignoring their statement altogether.]

JESSICA: Initially, I think, like most parents, we thought Alexis was just going through a phase. Her older brother went through the same school district and excelled in every way, and she really looks up to him. We thought maybe she was just thinking she had to be exactly like him: high grades, lots of friends, and able to get along with any and everyone. But over time, it seemed like her stress levels just got worse. All she ever talks about is not being "enough." Not smart enough, pretty enough, dressed up enough . . . it's constant and no matter how much we try to affirm her, nothing helps! When I brought up the topic of talking to a therapist with my mother, she said that all Alexis needs is time. I agreed. Maybe it was just a phase, but now it is affecting her grades.

MARK: One of our concerns was finding the right person to be the right fit for her if she did, in fact, need a therapist. We searched so many sites and asked for recommendations, and it's daunting because we didn't even know what we were looking for. And there's so many versions of therapists: PhDs, PsyDs, LPC, LCSW, MFT, etc. It just was overwhelming, so we decided to let it go and see if things would calm down. Also, neither of us have been in therapy, and we didn't want her to feel like something was wrong with her. Being one of the few Black kids at her school already creates a feeling of being "different" for her, and we were worried that telling Alexis we want her to be in therapy would just add to her feeling like she is different in yet another way. She tends to think in extremes like that.

THERAPIST: That makes sense that you use some caution about approaching this topic with her and even in your search to find the right clinician. And, Jessica, it sounds like you had the sounding board of your mother to help you figure out if it was the right time to even start therapy. [Validation of the described barriers without feeling compelled to dismiss or dispel the parents' concerns.] This is very helpful to hear because it gives me insight into how Alexis might be feeling about even participating in treatment now, feeling different and worried if coming to therapy means that something is wrong with her. [By reflecting back what was said, the therapist is creating an environment where the clients can speak freely, even if their candor is also an expression of their reticence about being there in the first place.]

JESSICA: Exactly. Therapy is still very taboo and for kids as young as her, we don't want to be looked at as the parents who didn't help their child or had too much pride to get her in therapy. But there is a part of us that does feel guilty that we are here. The world is tough enough, especially for Black people, and now on top of that, the anxiety and stress.

THERAPIST: Jessica, I really appreciate you bringing that up. It sounds like your hesitancy was a combination of things such as the taboo around mental health treatment seeking, wanting to help her and worrying if therapy was the right thing . . . and then just the upsetting reality of having these issues on top of what can be everyday experiences for Black people in our world. [Here, the therapist is demonstrating awareness of the barriers, linking the client's mentions of "taboo" to a typical thought process for Black clients. In doing so, this helps the client to feel both validated and safe to share more.] What you both are describing is very consistent with what our field is still trying to grapple with—how to reduce the stigma of mental health challenges and how to understand the impact of culture so that we can learn about and better support our clients. Being able to have open conversations like we are having is a great place to start. I am so glad that, in spite of all that, you are here. . . .

In Jessica's last statement, she is bringing up the ultimate barrier for many Black clients coming into therapy. She is describing how her child's stress and anxiety are exacerbating what is already a preexisting, ever-present stressor—being a Black person in spaces where she is the only one, in a world that makes it tougher. The therapist's interactions (e.g., reflective listening, Socratic questioning, unconditional positive regard) with the client are not novel; these are basic questioning and rapport-building strategies every therapist learns in their training. But when issues of race and worries about treatment seeking are raised by the client, does the therapist shy away from reflecting *those* types of statements? Clients are picking up on what therapists will and won't reflect, and for many therapists, *they* can become a treatment barrier if they are unwilling to talk about the issues relevant to their client's distress, including the topics of racism and discrimination.

Facilitators for Mental Health Treatment-Seeking for Black Clients

For clinicians to be able to create a welcoming and psychologically safe treatment experience for Black clients, they must be aware of the facilitators for treatment seeking. These efforts should include targeted continuing education requirements for training focused on culture, systemic racism in the history of the field of psychological services, and related topics, and considerations of how to better integrate these topics into the training of graduate students in psychology to better prepare them to work with Black clients.

This is not intended to be a sweeping generalization for all Black clients who may come into treatment. Research has shown that treatment facilitators for Black clients include having a support system, positive experiences in past treatment, and adequate follow-up. Each of these concepts is tied to the powerful role that community and connection play for Black families (Ayalon & Alvidrez, 2007).

Another facilitator for Black clients involves increased access to providers who may have some understanding of their lived experiences. The websites Therapy for Black Girls and Melanin and Mental Health, and the one for *Psychology Today* magazine, offer directories where potential clients may find clinicians who share an aspect of their identity that may help them feel that, at a minimum, there will be some ability to understand the shared lived experience of being Black in America. These sites also help clients prescreen for clinicians who accept their insurance or whose rates are affordable. Additionally, therapists on these directory sites share what presenting problems they treat, the type of treatment they provide, their philosophies on therapy and the process, and include pictures of themselves and links to their websites. For Black clients who may be reticent to seek services for fear that they might not be understood or that there a cultural divide would exist, these directory sites can help quell initial concerns. For a site like the one for *Psychology Today*, where clinicians of all backgrounds have profiles, clinicians who are not Black but hope to convey their intention and ability to talk about race and culture, should consider including statements in their profile that communicate such information.

For so many Black clients, the first step in identifying a clinician may include finding someone who can understand some basic aspects of their culture without having to explain and educate. However, Blackness is not a monolith, so it is critical that all clinicians have enough cultural humility to be open and willing to be curious about how environmental factors like racism and discrimination may be affecting the lives of their Black clients. In the earlier case example in this chapter, the family has indicated that their child is one of the few Black students in her school. If such information has been shared, there is likely a reason for it that could be explored by a clinician. If it isn't shared, a clinician should still deem it important to ask about the school climate and culture to be able to gain more understanding of the child's experience that has brought her to treatment. For Black clients, the perception of therapy and belief that a clinician is willing to connect and understand are what may help to facilitate treatment engagement for anyone but are especially meaningful for them (Scharff et al., 2021; Cabral & Smith, 2011).

In addition to the ease of finding a provider as a facilitator, the means to pay for one is also a big consideration. There are generous nonprofit organizations that help to subsidize therapy payments for Black clients seeking treatment and continue to reduce the barriers and stigma associated with mental health treatment seeking. Although there have been vast improvements in insurance coverage for mental health services, many clinicians in private practice may decide not to offer in-network services for various reasons. It is therefore important for those clinicians to alternatively consider how they might support their clients in getting reimbursements for services rendered (e.g., providing appropriate paperwork, helping with billing submission) or simply explaining to clients why they are not in network. For example:

"I want to explain to you why I am not currently participating in any insurance networks and my clients pay out of pocket and submit for reimbursement on their own. Many insurers may have specific requirements for reimbursement that would include specific diagnoses. It is my sense that sometimes the diagnostic manuals we rely on do not always capture the stressors and life challenges that might bring a person to therapy. While I know that you are expressing that your daughter is experiencing what sounds like anxiety, and I would likely indicate that as a general diagnosis, the insurance company might have expectations about the length of time they may be willing to cover such a diagnosis and may want supporting documentation to justify covering it. I also believe that some of your daughter's stress may be—based on what you have shared—linked to race-based stress. As one of very few Black students in her school and the kinds of remarks and microaggressions that she has been experiencing may better account for why she is anxious and feeling tremendous pressure to perform perfectly. These are the types of considerations that are, unfortunately, not captured by our field's current diagnostic tools. I also choose to help my clients collect their out-of-network benefit or use a sliding scale so that those barriers and administrative issues do not prevent us from working together. What questions do you have for me about this?"

Again, in this example, it is the transparency, openness, and opportunity for the client to ask more questions that may help create more engagement in treatment. Therapy is still a mystery to many people who have only learned about it from TV or books. For Black clients, their often healthy cultural suspicion in seeking treatment means that therapists should be transparent and focused on demystifying the therapeutic process from the very beginning of services. In the therapist's explanation above, there is clear acknowledgment of the limitations within our field in the recognition of the impact of race and discrimination on the life of the client. Moreover, the therapist is leaning into the fact that this limitation is part of why they choose not to participate in insurance. In the case where the therapist does take insurance, there would also need to be a conversation about what that exactly means and what information will be shared. This will help the client understand the types of documentation that insurers may need or ask for, and be able to truly make an informed consent to services if they are seeing a provider in network. In this chapter, we explored how to routinely consider the barriers and facilitators when selecting therapeutic interventions. In Part II, which focuses on parents and community, we discuss how to implement them in a culturally humble manner.

CHAPTER TAKEAWAYS

- Increased awareness and acknowledgment of the impact of racism and discrimination on the mental health of Black clients are critical for all clinicians to understand. And since there are significantly fewer therapists of color in the field of mental health—particularly among psychologists—understanding the barriers and facilitators for Black clients should lead to adaptations of standard therapeutic practices that will help with engagement, connection, and improve the overall experience for Black clients.

- Clinicians do not have to reinvent the wheel but can use tried-and-true therapeutic techniques to increase their own comfort with discussing issues of race and discrimination, rather than relying on clients to act on their own in bringing the relevance of those issues into the therapeutic space.

CHAPTER 4

Preparing the Next Generation
Culturally Responsive Supervision

> Education is our passport to the future, for tomorrow belongs to the people who prepare for it today.
> —MALCOLM X (1964)

Terry is an African American cisgender female doctoral psychology student working in an intensive outpatient program for clients presenting with dual diagnoses. Most of the clients served in the program are young adults, representing mostly Black and Latino communities. Terry's supervisor, a white cisgender female clinician, has been working in this program for 10 years and has a great deal of experience dealing with this population. Most services are provided in a group format, and Terry has been cofacilitating a group that consists of group members with a dual diagnosis of substance dependence and a serious mental illness or mood disorder. Terry comes into supervision with some questions about the previous group and one of the participants, named Kat. Kat is a 24-year-old African American woman who has been attending group for several weeks. She occasionally participates but usually has low energy and needs much coaxing to participate. When she does, she sometimes annoys other participants because they claim she complains too much and never tries any of the recommendations made to her by the cotherapists or participants:

TERRY: I noticed that yesterday, Kat seemed very animated and her energy was very different than usual. She actually was more engaged and helpful to other group members. I was wondering if you think it may be good for me to chat with her about how she has been implementing her coping skills and see if maybe her treatment plan could be updated?

SUPERVISOR: I noticed that, too, but I was also struck by her hair. It was very different. She seems to change her hair very frequently but yesterday, it was pretty wild, wasn't it?

TERRY: I didn't really notice because she changes it all the time.

SUPERVISOR: I know that sometimes, when people are entering into a manic phase, they may make wild, unusual decisions from the more serious to the more mundane. It may be nothing, but that wild hair, the shirt she chose to wear . . . what did it say? "Good Trouble." Clearly, she was letting us know what she came to do in the group—stir the pot and bring all that overly animated energy in to throw off the flow of the group.

TERRY: I took it to be a reference to the phrase "good trouble" that John Lewis talked about when he was living. (*silence*) The one about getting into good trouble to fight for civil rights?

SUPERVISOR: Oh wow, I didn't even know about that, and honestly, I doubt she did either! She doesn't seem like the type that would even know who John Lewis was. I thought she was kind of being mischievous by wearing it. She is diagnosed with bipolar disorder, and when bipolar patients are in a manic phase, you sometimes see them wear their hair in wild styles all over their head, extra make-up, attention-seeking clothes, etc.

TERRY: Well, her hair is just in an afro. It looks like she took out her braids and just let her hair go natural instead of wearing braids as usual. But about her increased energy and better contributions in group . . .

In this vignette, there are a few notable interactions between Terry and the supervisor. The racial identity of a supervisor and their supervisee can impact some or all of the supervisory experience, particularly when the client's racial identity is central to their presenting problem in therapy. In this cross-cultural supervisory interaction, there are a few moments where the supervisee is in the position of explaining to her supervisor alternative and/or neutral explanations for the client's appearance and behaviors. While the supervisor is in an authoritative role and has experience working in the clinical setting and with the populations served there, it is evident that they may lack awareness of subtle cultural expressions demonstrated by the client. The hairstyle changes and the message on the shirt alerted the supervisor to possible manifestations of whatever the mental health issue was, whereas for Terry, she did not consider them at all in her assessment because she viewed those same indicators as just being a part of Black culture. Had Terry's supervisor also been a Black clinician, would they have made the same assessment as Terry? While cultures are not monolithic and have nuances, it is possible that Terry may not have had to explain things to the same extent if she had had a supervisor who shared her same racial background (and thus understood some of the references seen in the client's presentation). That supervisor may not have even bothered pointing them out if they were perceived as having no bearing on the client's clinical issues, but rather a general expression of their culture.

In this chapter, culturally responsible supervision is discussed with the understanding that, as stated in previous chapters, much of the workforce in the behavioral health field consists of white professionals. The result is that cross-cultural supervision dyads with a white supervisor occurs more frequently. In discussing culturally responsive supervision, the aim is to help supervisors—regardless of their racial or cultural identity—to consider their own culture and that of their supervisees in a meaningful way to cultivate opportunities for both parties to learn and apply culturally appropriate treatment.

The Role of a Supervisor

The role of a supervisor in any field is one that requires leadership skills, availability, expertise in specific subject matters, emotional intelligence, and a willingness to continue to learn and stay abreast of the innovations of their respective fields. Supervisors are inherently held to a certain standard by their supervisees,[1] and this *relationship* can be crucial in shaping the developing workforce. Supervisors in the field of psychology are expected to carry out not just the priorities

1. Enhance the professional competence of the trainee.
2. Enhance science-informed practice.
3. Monitor the quality of services provided.
4. Protect the public.
5. Provide a gatekeeping function for entry into the profession.

This list captures the overarching ideals of the role of the psychologist as supervisor, and contained within each item are plenty of tasks, goals, and objectives to accomplish these goals. While the goals seem relatively straightforward, they are multifaceted. In recent years in the United States and abroad, the landscape of our field has significantly shifted in terms of the cultural and political impact on mental health in daily life. Recall from our discussion in Chapter 3 that broad events and issues in society can have a profound effect on a Black person's sense of security and safety, even if they are not directly involved in those events. The COVID-19 pandemic; the murder of George Floyd, Breonna Taylor, and other unarmed Black people at the hands of law enforcement; the continued political strife associated with the 2020 U.S. presidential election; and the subsequent insurrection at the U.S. Capitol in Washington, D.C., are just a few of the many events that have had a significant impact on the sense of safety, health, and well-being of many people. But more than that, these issues have had an impact on people's sense of belonging and ability to feel safe in a way that is strikingly different for this next generation of mental health providers to contend with. The collective experience we all have had cannot be understated, and for psychology supervisors, it behooves us to be aware of, and account for, how these issues have impacted the way supervisees will come into the field.

---

[1] The term "supervisee" will be used interchangeably in this chapter with "trainee" and "student." and policies of their agencies, but also the intentions set forth by the Board of Educational Affairs of the APA (Falender & Shafranske, 2021). According to these APA guidelines (APA, 2014), supervision is intended to:

As supervisors in the field of mental health, it is imperative that we move beyond cultural competence. We must transition to being more responsive and impactful in our supervision and create a space where our supervisees can talk about how their cultures, the cultures of those they serve, and the cultures of those they work for impact their work in many ways. As we have pointed out in earlier chapters, from how we diagnose, to what services we offer, to the policies we create in our systems, culture is the underlying thread that runs through these aspects of what we do. The application of cultural considerations in counseling professions arose in prominence in the mid-1990s, indicating that compared to the many years of this profession, exploration of how cultural issues are addressed in supervisory relationships is still relatively new. (Fukuyama, 1994). In order to engage in this type of supervision, we first have to gain a sense of where the field of psychology is and where supervisors tend to fall short.

How Supervisors Can Enhance Their Cultural Competency through Cultural Humility

Most supervisees of color are highly likely to be in a cross-cultural supervisory relationship. In 2022, 83% of U.S. psychologists identified as white, 4% as Asian, 7% as Latino, 3% as Black/African American, and 1% as multiracial (APA, 2022). These numbers indicated that the field of doctoral-level psychologists is not reflective of the general U.S. population with regard to race/ethnicity. While the rate of early-career psychologists representing minority race/ethnic groups has increased over the past decade, it is still true that most supervisees of graduate students in psychology are white.

Taking this into consideration, what does it mean for supervisors? Black students entering the field of psychology can go through multiple training experiences in their schooling and never encounter a supervisor who looks like them. But, should that matter? If a student is interested in learning about cognitive-behavioral treatment or wants to work with populations with severe mental health challenges, should the race of the supervisor even matter? Wouldn't it be more important for the supervisor to know how to treat in this type of orientation, or that type of care setting? Does race really matter in the supervisory relationship when it comes to Black trainees or trainees of any race treating Black clients? In fact, yes, it does matter. And furthermore, the burden of ensuring the best possible supervisory experience lies in the supervisor's ability to understand and recognize all of this. Culturally responsive supervision can be a critical part of training that can ensure all trainees understand the value in ongoing self-reflection of the self they bring to any interaction, the humility to recognize hidden spots and correct for that, and the empathy to connect with their trainees in ways that both educate and empower them to be successful with their clients.

Culturally responsive supervision (CRS) relates to the goal of reducing the risk of exacerbating race-based traumatic stress in Black supervisees as well as in Black clients receiving psychological services from supervisees of any race. Most models of supervision place an emphasis on the cultural competence of a supervisee, and not as much on the supervisor's level of competence. The focus on "competence" is one that the field should shift away from for a few reasons. Cultural competence is often identified as having the ability to appreciate and interact with people of differing cultures and belief systems, and has been one of the core competencies for psychological education for many years (DeAngelis, 2015). There is nothing inherently wrong with cultural competence, and it is a great place to start if we want to be able to know a little about a lot of different people. However, culturally responsive supervision—which is also sometimes referred to as multicultural supervision—takes this discussion about culture one step further. A core concept within CRS is being aware of what one does NOT know and being curious enough about that to humbly engage with a supervisee and be both teacher and learner. While cultural competence encourages one to become knowledgeable about different cultures, culturally responsive supervision encourages one to recognize that it is not possible to know about every culture, and that even in getting to know more, we still see what we learn through the lens of our own culture. CRS helps us to be accepting, rather than embarrassed or insulted when a supervisee catches our **hidden spot**.[2] It

---

[2] In an effort to use culturally responsive language, "hidden spot" is used in place of what is typically called a "blind spot." The meaning—indicating that people may be unaware of their implicit biases or ignorance of certain cultural norms different than their own—is the same, but the term "hidden spots" will be used throughout the text.

also makes us less defensive when we have clearly engaged in a microaggression with one of our trainees.

Hook and colleagues (Hook et al., 2013) defined cultural humility as "the ability to maintain an interpersonal stance of openness to another regarding aspects of cultural identities" (p. 353). It is a key component of providing CRS as it impacts our way of being with our supervisees. Supervisors who practice cultural humility are both willing AND committed to self-examination. Greene-Moten and Minkler (2020) discuss how embracing a "both/and" mentality as it relates to cultural competence and cultural humility can collectively facilitate self-reflection and increased awareness on the part of providers, creating space for learning. I can recall many times as a psychology trainee encountering white supervisors who minimized the role of race in how I understood a client's behavior or statements, or that made me question my own *lived experience* of racial differences in the presentation of client coping skills as being pathological in some way. For the few that I encountered, I feel confident in saying that their *intentions* were likely not to dismiss me or cause harm. They probably felt as if they were teaching me and helping me become an astute clinician, not falling prey to racial stereotypes to explain client presentation or using my own experiences to project my own beliefs onto my clients. But the *impact* was a feeling of doubt in my own abilities as an early trainee. For so many Black students in psychology, there is no one else who looks like them in their graduate school cohort, or in their externship settings—many of which are housed in communities that are usually serving diverse communities of individuals who do share their race/ethnicity.

Black psychology trainees and colleagues have often shared their perspectives and experiences with me, saying things like:

"I don't feel like I belong here."
"Major imposter syndrome. I feel like I am constantly trying to convince people that I should be here."
"It's exhausting being the only one at the proverbial table."
"My supervisor commented on my hair . . . again!"

For supervisors, microaggressions seem to be one of the most common offenses that are reported. Derald Wing Sue and his colleagues identified the term "racial microaggressions" and defined it as brief indignities that can be verbal, behavioral, or environmental, and that communicate hostile or derogatory slights toward people of color (Sue et al., 2007). These slights do not have to be intentional, and that is directly germane to culturally responsive supervision. The *intention* of a statement or supervisory interaction is less important than the *impact* that it has on the supervisee.

Cultural Humility: Working on Being Reflective and Responsive

Ashley and Lipscomb (2018) found that supervisors often overestimate how reflective and responsive they are with supervisees when it comes to the practices of cultural humility. Though their research was in graduate study in the field of education, it is likely similar across any field where supervision is a crucial element for trainees. In their work, when asking both supervisors and supervisees if supervisors take on the role as learner, supervisors responded that they do assume that position, while supervisees stated that supervisors do not because they are in a position of leadership and privilege. Furthermore, many supervisee respondents reported that supervisors rarely talk about issues such as power, privilege, or intersectionality (having more than one minority identity in one individual, such as being Black and a woman). When supervisors do talk about these topics, it is often in reference to clients and not about the supervisee's identity.

Other studies echo this sentiment. Black supervisees describe feelings of invalidation and reluctance to share their clinical conceptualizations related to race, for fear of how it will be received by their supervisors who do not share their racial identity (Constantine & Sue, 2007). Supervisees of color have also identified "culturally unresponsive" supervision as behaviors where supervisors ignored, dismissed, or minimized the impact of culture in the client's situation. One study reported that trainees in these supervisory relationships reduced their disclosures during supervision meetings as a result of this repeated minimization of the impact of culture on their clinical work (Burkard et al., 2006). The risk of culturally unresponsive supervision is that trainees, particularly those who identify as Black or African American, may feel supervision is not a safe place to talk about the role of race in their experiences and those of their clients. This means they are not able to access the meaningful learning experiences that are the building blocks of who they will be as psychologists. Falender et al. (2014) also discuss the importance of the supervisor reflecting on how their own assumptions and values—often influenced by culture—can help them in their efforts to maintain cultural humility.

As mentioned in Chapter 2, Sandeen, Moore, and Swanda (2018) discuss the concept of RLP, which is an approach that allows us to seamlessly layer a culturally responsive and humble lens, whether we are engaged in direct service or in a supervisory or teaching role. As part of this practice in supervision, a first step is to consider our own "bias spots." The authors describe *hot*, *hidden*, and *soft* spots as areas of bias practitioners and supervisors should reflect on to reduce the risk of engaging in culturally insensitive practice. These "spots" are inextricably linked to aspects of our identity and how we perceive our own power and privilege related to them. A hot spot is a bias we may possess that results in significant emotional distress when we experience something that we believe is connected to one of our identities that is deemed powerless or oppressed. In the example of Terry and her supervisor, a potential hot spot is that Terry shares the same racial identity as her client. The supervisor's assessment of the client's cultural expression through her hair and attire could have resulted in Terry feeling uncomfortable, or even angry, about the supervisor's lack of understanding and the ease of making the client's cultural expression some indicator of pathology. Thus, the shared cultural identity with a client can make a clinician or supervisor vulnerable to experiencing discomfort and distress on behalf of the client. A hidden spot (see footnote 2 above) is a bias that may often be outside of our awareness because it relates to our lack of recognition or lack of sensitivity to identities that we do not share with others. Or, we may be unaware of it because our own power and privilege interfere with our recognizing the different experience of others. A good example of a hidden spot can be seen when someone with a privileged identity makes a comment about a purchase they are considering, along the lines of

"It's not a lot of money, just a few hundred bucks." Making such a comment suggests a lack of awareness that there are many people for whom a few hundred dollars is an exorbitant amount. Finally, soft spots are places where a supervisor is at risk for overidentifying or being overly sympathetic to a client or supervisee. The result is setting a low bar of expectations due to sharing an identity or overconfidence in their own understanding of the client's or supervisee's identity, power, or privilege. An example of a soft spot in action could be those times a clinician decides not to address when a Black client avoids engaging in therapy strategies in between sessions because of their belief that the world is hard enough on Black people. The clinician does not want to add to the weight that they believe the Black client is already carrying. A clinician in this case is acting with good intent, but the overall impact is that it can be patronizing to act in a manner that holds Black clients to a lower standard in their therapy engagement. In strange ways, a soft spot may reaffirm stereotypes about Black clients by not setting the same expectations of them as any other client.

Soft spots are explained in the RLP model as being triggered if and when a clinician has some level of awareness of marginalized identities and how they are affected by discrimination and bias. As a result, that clinician may make assumptions about the client based on some aspect of their identity and lower their expectations in an effort to alleviate some of that systemic stress. The impact of having a soft spot in a clinical relationship is that the clinician may not empower the client to practice the challenging strategies in treatment. An example of this that often occurs is when practitioners make assumptions about what clients can do if they have a cognitive impairment and limit the rigor of treatment in a way that disempowers them.

The RLP model applies these "spots" to the clinician–client dyad, but in our application of it to the supervisor–supervisee dyad (or even the supervisor–supervisee–client triad), the experiencing of these hot, soft, and hidden spots could occur based on differing aspects of shared identity. If Terry was a white clinician treating a Black client and the supervisor was also Black, perhaps the supervisor would be at risk of experiencing a hot spot due to identifying with the client because of their shared race.

How Supervision Should Work

In the vignette opening this chapter, we see what could be viewed as a few of these microaggressions that occur simply because the supervisor jumped to conclusions about the client's mental health status, as opposed to asking questions first. In this case, a hidden spot is illustrated by the supervisor. When Terry began to discuss Kat's behavioral changes in group, the supervisor began to talk about Kat's hair and clothes. The supervisor is not making statements that could be labeled as overly racist or racially insensitive. But the supervisor clearly has a few hidden spots. In recent years, especially following George Floyd's murder in 2020, the phrase "good trouble" began to rise in prominence, particularly among the Black community. The words—tweeted by civil rights icon and former congressman John Lewis in 2018—referred to his call to action for people to get into "good trouble, necessary trouble, and help redeem the soul of America." That phrase moved through social media and is known to many. To those who may not be aware of Lewis and his work, a shirt that says "Good Trouble" could easily be misconstrued. But such does not have to be the response if one simply practiced culturally responsive supervision.

What would CRS look like in the interaction with Terry? Perhaps the supervisor could have been curious instead of accusatorial:

> "I saw Kat was wearing a shirt that said 'Good Trouble.' What do you think that means? I thought maybe it was a message for us, but I could be wrong. What do you think?"

But even if the supervisor did not catch herself the first time, what could she have said after Terry referenced the John Lewis quote?

> "I hadn't even considered that! Maybe that was it. If that is the case, that could be a good way to start a conversation with her in an individual session since that phrase might mean something to her and maybe even motivates her to get the most out of the group. What do you think?"

Notice the cadence in these two alternative reactions. The supervisor is not completely abandoning what her initial reactions were, but is open to further exploring this subject and considering Terry's hypothesis that Kat's wearing the shirt may reflect her being inspired by the phrase "good trouble," and nothing sinister in nature. The other benefit to this alternative flow of discussion is that it elevates Terry to the role of teacher and the supervisor to the role of student—albeit for a few seconds. This is another critical element of culturally responsive supervision—a moment to model humility in the supervisor–supervisee relationship. It is in these moments when the supervisee becomes a teacher, which helps to build their sense of competency about what they know and their ability to teach it to others in a collaborative way.

For better or for worse, supervision sets the tone for how the trainee develops and sets out in the clinical world as a provider. For Black trainees and for trainees who are treating Black clients, it is imperative that supervisors make room for discussions that can be uncomfortable, even humbling, but collaborative. Supervisors who don't make the effort to establish relationships in which supervisees feel safe raising such issues miss an opportunity to work effectively with Black trainees. And, in fact, they risk becoming part of a cycle of racial trauma that results in work environments that feel unresponsive at best, and unsafe and even toxic at worst.

Where Do I Start?

Explore and Talk about Identity

Hays (2001) created a phenomenal framework that simply allows people to consider their many identities. She refers to it as the ADDRESSING framework, one that comprises a range of identities people hold: age, developmental disabilities, religion, ethnic and racial identity, socioeconomic status, sexual orientation, indigenous heritage, national origin, and gender. One place to start as a supervisor would be to consider the identities in this framework most salient to you and your worldview as a mental health professional. This is the lens you bring to the work. Then consider your supervisee's identities, or better yet, ask them to share theirs with you once you have established a rapport with them. If you share any identities, what are some of the variations you have with your supervisee in how you believe your shared identities differ in terms of worldview. This allows you as the supervisor to learn from your trainee and for them to appreciate your recognition that no identity category is monolithic in nature. This can be a great rapport-building strategy early on as you establish your roles in the supervisory dyad.

The ADDRESSING framework can also be helpful as an ongoing reference tool for discussing client differences as well. In the vignette above, we know a few things about Kat's identity. We know she identifies as a woman (gender), she is African American (race/ethnicity), she is 24 years old so we know at the time of this writing (2022), she was born in the late 1990s (age, generational influence). Supervisory meetings could include discussion of what types of messages Kat received about mental illness growing up as a Black child in the early 2000s and 2010s. Is there anything about the individuals in the group and their identities that may cause her to usually be more withdrawn and what changed that made her become more open and energetic in the recent group?

Try not to allow your own anxiety about making errors in these types of discussions to prevent you from discussing them at all. In the book *So You Want to Talk about Race* (2019), Ijeoma Oluo identifies what white people can do if conversations about race go wrong. Among the solutions are behavioral strategies that are relatively simple, such as simply apologizing for the error, not beating oneself up, and taking the risk and committing to trying to have the conversation again.

Let's say that the conversation between Terry and her supervisor about Kat ended exactly as originally written. Now, Terry has walked away from the situation believing that the supervisor's focus on only limited details about Kat indicated her ignorance of Black cultural forms of expression and normative hair styles, and thus a hidden spot about the meaning of Kat's improved engagement in group. Let's say the supervisor recognized this error and wanted to address it the next day. Here, is how she might approach that:

> "Terry, I was sharing my thoughts with another colleague yesterday about Kat and after talking with them, I realized I misread some of Kat's presentation in group yesterday. I just want to apologize to you for that. I know you were trying to explain, and I think since I am

not as familiar with African American culture and the nuances of certain forms of expression of cultural norms from that lens, I definitely got ahead of myself—or maybe in my own way—yesterday. In the future, please feel free to let me know if I step into that hidden spot again. I have been doing this so long that I sometimes get stuck on seeing everything as part of a person's mental health diagnosis and that's where your fresh set of eyes could be really helpful in our supervision meetings."

Again, it is not about saying the right thing or perfectly phrasing everything. Also, it may not even be about actually understanding or agreeing with your supervisee or their interpretation of the client's behavior. The CRS approach is more about being willing to share where you have a hidden spot, acknowledging the offense, and opening yourself up to doing better in the future to reduce risk and engage in more collaboration with your trainee about their clients.

How Do I Improve My Skills?

Do the Work While No One Is Watching

To borrow a sports metaphor, people tend to play how they practice. In order to be culturally responsive, one should consider using as many opportunities as possible to practice having conversations with people about culture, cultural differences, stereotypes, and paying attention to calling out when they encounter microaggressions or racially insensitive or violent behaviors when such situations do occur. When I train professionals in CRS, I tend to mention that a good benchmark on how far along you are in this journey is how you act when you are *not* in the supervisory dyad. For example, say you are at a family gathering, and comments are made about racial minority groups, or your good friend posts something insensitive about a racial group on social media. Can you notice that and call it for what it is (at least to yourself)? The more experience you have in practicing the skill of noticing microaggressions, exploring your own identities, and continuing to educate yourself, the more you will be able to naturally and authentically engage in these practices in your capacity as a supervisor. Taking a culturally responsive approach to your life means you acknowledge that *everyone* has a culture and identities that are salient to them in different contexts. The practice of self-awareness helps us to be more open and sensitive to the salient identities of others. Upshaw et al. (2020) also recommends dialoguing with people of other cultures, continuing education, and using mentorship as other ways to engage in internal work to better meet the needs of supervisees.

Be Reflective of Yourself and Practice with Your Supervisees

The RLP model calls for supervisors and practitioners to engage in each of its components. This can mean that as supervisors, we must reflect on our own identities (the use of the ADDRESSING framework is a good start) and also think about what aspects of our identities come with power, privilege, history of or current oppression, or are neutral in nature. We can also take time to look for the aforementioned bias spots that we may have. The "local" component of this framework calls for us to be aware of the culture, broadly speaking, of the communities we serve. We should consider not just the population demographics, but that of our supervisees, and what is occurring within the general context of the mental health landscape. An example of this is developing an understanding of how the COVID-19 pandemic may have changed the trends in mental health presentation in clients and its impact on the training experiences of supervisees in graduate school cohorts spanning the acute phases of the pandemic. The "practice" component is to regularly engage in learning and activities that offer us opportunities to deepen our cultural awareness.

Create Brave Spaces

The concept of bravery is simple: One must be scared to possess bravery. Talking about race in cross-cultural dyads or groups can be scary for all involved. But for Black clients and trainees, the discussion of race is not unfamiliar. Groups that have been historically oppressed and marginalized have been talking about the treatment they receive based simply on their race or other marginalized identity for ages. What may be new is having someone who is not from that same background express genuine interest in understanding how race shapes the way a supervisee will approach their work in the mental health field. Supervisors set the tone for when and how those conversations occur, and the more open they are to hearing the experiences of supervisees, the more connected they may feel, which could lead to a richer, more meaningful learning experience for both parties. This is slightly different than the commonly used phrase of a "safe space." Safe spaces tend to be interpreted as those where anything can be said and there will be no pushback, judgment, or call to action.

CHAPTER TAKEAWAYS

- Culturally responsive supervision (CRS) is a comprehensive term that encompasses cultural humility, cultural competence, multicultural supervisory approaches, and RLP as a guide for supervision.

- The success of CRS implementation begins with a willingness on the part of the supervisor to be self-reflective of their own culture and use frameworks such as Hays's ADDRESSING model to begin to explore their own salient identities that may contribute to their biases.

- Culturally responsive supervisors are willing to function in the role of both teacher AND student. They create opportunities in the supervisory experience for exploration of the impact of cultural identities in the supervisee–client interaction, as the supervisory experience often is paralleled in the client's experience with their therapist.

- Leading with curiosity is often the best approach. For Black supervisees, the research has shown that they often feel as if the power differential in the supervisory relationship prevents them from disclosing information to their supervisor if they feel that person is unwilling to ask them about aspects of culture. Making assumptions can lead to reinforcing that reticence to share, which ultimately impacts the clients they are serving. Supervisors should ask questions, as in the case example above about the client's shirt.

- Practice when no one is watching, and in this case, "no one" means when your supervisees are not around. Your supervisory meetings should not be the only time when you discuss issues relevant to culture. Use time with others in your life to explore and discuss culture to build your comfort and ability to engage in what can sometimes be an uncomfortable discourse. Remember that culture is tied to so much of what we do, what foods we eat, how we dress, and so forth. There are plenty of opportunities to practice these skills and build your capacity for creating and encouraging brave spaces to talk about race.

PART II
RACIAL TRAUMA IN COMMUNITY SETTINGS

CHAPTER 5

Pen or Pencil
Addressing Racial Trauma in Schools

> When children attend schools that place a greater value on discipline and security than on knowledge and intellectual development, they are attending prep schools for prison.
> —ANGELA DAVIS (2003)[1]

Brian is a 15-year-old Black male student who is repeating the 9th grade at a school that is majority-Black, and has embedded law enforcement and metal detectors. He is not keeping up and is performing poorly in most of his classes. His best grades are a B in creative writing and a B in music appreciation. His teachers in these subjects describe Brian as "an absolute delight to work with," while his math teacher says that he seems distracted and "in another world" and "defiant." His teachers indicate that Brian does not disrupt class, although he is often found doodling, cannot remember instructions, and often asks teachers to repeat them. They say Brian works best one-to-one but will not stay for extra tutoring sessions after school. He seems overwhelmed by assignments and has great difficulty organizing his work.

Brian readily admits that he finds it difficult to pay attention and daydreams or sleeps in class. He says he has no idea how to study for a

---

[1] Excerpt from Angela Y. Davis, "Slavery, Civil Rights, and Abolitionist Perspectives Toward Prison" from *Are Prisons Obsolete?* Copyright © 2003 by Angela Y. Davis. Reprinted with the permission of The Permissions Company, LLC on behalf of Seven Stories Press, sevenstories.com.

test, does not "get" what he is reading, and becomes lost when he tries to reread passages. He likes his creative writing teacher, a heavyset African American woman who reminds him of his mom. He wishes he did better in her class because he wants her to like him. Yesterday, he learned that she is leaving the school to teach at a charter school. He says that she is probably tired of working with delinquents and wants to work with kids who can learn.

The impact of racial trauma on young people starts—or is best avoided—in the classroom. Clinicians working in school systems have the unique opportunity to educate, advocate, and intervene in a meaningful way that can disrupt the effects of racial trauma. This chapter examines the influence racial trauma has on the **achievement gap** and school discipline practices, all of which contribute to the **school-to-prison pipeline**.

Who Is Teaching Black Youth?

During the 2020–2021 school year, white teachers made up 80% of 3.8 million full-time and part-time public schoolteachers (National Center for Education Statistics [NCES], 2023). In schools where most students are Black, on average, two-thirds of the teachers identify as white non-Hispanic (Spiegelman, 2020). Efforts to improve representation in teaching so far have been insufficient, despite the well-documented benefit of Black students having diverse teachers (El-Mekki, 2021). According to the Government Accountability Office (GAO; Nowicki, 2022), schools in the United States remain divided among racial, ethnic, and economic lines, even as the K–12 population grows more diverse. In the 2020–2021 school year, approximately 18.5 million children (more than a third of students in America) attended schools in which 75% or more of the students were of a single race or ethnicity. The GAO attributes this lack of diversity in schools to district boundaries determining which school a student can attend; these boundaries continue to be drawn along racial and ethnic lines.

Many of the approximately 80% of white teachers in the United States find themselves in a cultural context different from their own. Black students are twice as likely as their white peers to attend schools in high-poverty areas, schools that are underresourced, and schools where teacher tenure is lowest (Garcia, 2020). One cost of this disparity is a racially traumatic pattern of non-Black teachers who are not adequately prepared to teach Black students.

Teacher preparation programs too often fall short of giving new teachers culturally responsive techniques for working with Black youth. There is a long-recognized need for interculturally competent teachers. However, many teachers still feel ill-prepared in working with culturally diverse populations (Romijn, Slot, & Leseman, 2021). This lack of preparation can lead to a gross underestimation of Black students' academic abilities (Will, 2020), which can have far-reaching consequences (i.e., achievement, discipline, graduation rate gaps).

While we wait for teacher education programs to catch up and adequately prepare our newest teachers to work with diverse populations, especially our Black youth, clinicians can play a key role in highlighting and addressing these issues with teachers and administrators. School psychologists, guidance counselors, school-based social workers, and other counseling professionals can not only set an example but also *be* the example. Clinicians can speak of liberation and **equity** for Black students, and they can provide students with the tools to secure it. For example, clinicians can explore their own personal knowledge, beliefs, and attitudes about working with Black students. Then, clinicians can work to ensure that each Black student has access to a school counseling program that advocates specifically for them in addition to all students (American School Counselor Association [ASCA], 2021). Moreover, on an administrative leave, clinicians can advocate for Black students by challenging and changing racially traumatic guidelines, policies, practices, and procedures.

The Clinician in the School

There may be many different forms of clinicians in the schools, including the school psychologist, school social worker, school guidance counselor or school counselor. The clinician is a backstage figure in the school who can advocate for Black students facing race-based traumatic stress. Even more importantly, the clinician can foster healing from racial trauma, which is often part of Black students' experience. Advocacy for Black students comes in many forms. One way clinicians can help mitigate disparities within school discipline is by assisting teachers with techniques to build better relationships with their Black students. One example is to have curious conversations by which a teacher can open the doors of opportunity for Black students to speak on their experience and culture. Another way to foster relations is to seek feedback from the Black students. Regardless of race, it is impossible for teachers to fully understand the experiences of Black students, unless they directly ask their Black students. Just implementing these two ideas can increase the connection between a teacher and their Black students.

Professional guidance is especially important for Black students whose teachers find building positive relationships difficult (Okonofua, Walton, & Eberhardt, 2016). Clinicians can consult with teachers to sharpen their skills, such as in recognizing that Black children are not a monolith. Through knowing their students as individuals, teachers can celebrate what they bring to the classroom—and enjoy a more genuine connection with their students.

One technique the clinician can use is to assist teachers in building insight into racial trauma and the link between Black student's experiences of being racially stigmatized and their psychological experience in school. For example, the constant threat of being sent out of class, detention, suspension, and even expulsion takes a toll on Black students. These threats are likely to limit their engagement in the classroom, which has been shown to increase the likelihood of poor standardized grades and even dropping out of school (Jones & Gregory, 2011). Create training for teachers highlighting this issue and educate them on ways to build rapport.

I (J. R. J.-D.) had the opportunity to work with an underserved school district with predominately Black students. There were a good number of Black teachers and teachers from marginalized backgrounds; about half the teachers and staff were white. I (J. R. J.-D.) created a training program for the teachers and staff centered on engaging students and meeting them where they were. In the presentation, we spoke about the curriculum reflecting the students' life and experiences. In order for that to happen, teachers would need to know the students' hobbies, music, family makeup and dynamics, and most importantly gain an understanding of the community in which the students are embedded.

Key to building rapport with Black students is getting to know them as individuals. Black students are not all the same. Learn how to pronounce their names correctly and be sure not to call a Black student by another Black student's name. According to Watts (2021), many students recall the experience of being called the name of another Black student in their class. This is a form of racial stress and can be harmful. A teacher calling a Black student by the wrong name can send the message that the teacher does not know who the student is or value them as an individual.

In many classrooms, conversations about the Black experience start from a place of struggle or pain. A Black male student once said that while he was in his high school psychology class, the teacher offered statistics about Black boys not graduating from high school and related that there were more Black men in jail and prison than in college. This student was one of two Black males in the class, and he sat there heartbroken and ashamed, feeling as if all his classmates' eyes were on him. The clinician can assist teachers like this by pressing them to present Black culture and history in ways that are affirming and not from a deficit model. Black students should be able to feel the same joy as others when their history or truth is spoken in the classroom.

Clinicians can also advocate for Black students by assisting school administration in reviewing policies that unfairly target Black students. What's important to know is that these policies do not target Black students explicitly on the surface. For example, some schools have dress code policies that inadvertently (or intentionally) target the cultural norms of Black students. Black students are sent home and suspended for not complying with hair "norms" that are part of dress codes. Some states have adopted the **Creating a Respectful and Open World for Natural Hair (CROWN) Act** to ban discrimination against natural hair, which unduly targets Black individuals. Although progress has been made, race-based hair discrimination remains a systemic problem in schools. Counselors can assist the administration with examining such data, such as data specific to the disproportionate effects of discipline policies. A 2011 landmark study conducted by the Council of State Governments in Texas demonstrated that 97% of the suspensions that occurred in the state were based on local policies or the discretionary decisions of local school officials (Schwarz, 2011). Black students were 31% more likely to be suspended or expelled based on those discretionary decisions than were white or Hispanic students (Schwarz, 2011). When clinicians highlight studies such as these, they are using data to drive the decisions and policies of their school district. Thanks to extensive training, school clinicians often have a foundational knowledge in research that teachers and administrators may not have and, therefore, can create studies and analyze data on a school or even at a district level.

Racial Trauma and the Achievement Gap

Racial trauma shows up in many ways in schools. One way is how it contributes to the achievement gap. The achievement gap is defined as the disparities in educational achievement between differing racial groups (NCES, 2024). The result of the racial achievement gap is that Black students are more likely to receive lower grades, score lower on standardized tests, not graduate from high school, and are less likely to pursue, enter, and complete college than their white counterparts (U.S. Department of Education [USDOE], 2020). The consequences of this gap are far-reaching. According to the Department of Education, the racial achievement gap leads to lower earnings, poor health, and higher rates of incarceration (Bradley, 2022).

The Black/white achievement gap occurs when white students outperform Black students and the difference in the average scores for these two groups is statistically significant. There are many influences and causes for this gap, such as school segregation by race and poverty (Startz, 2020), parental education attainment (Assari et al., 2021), **structural racism** (Merolla & Jackson, 2019), and economic status (Howard, 2016). These are all strong predictors of the racial achievement gap; however, here, we will specifically look at the impact of racial trauma.

Racial trauma is not a new phenomenon, but its visibility has increased due to social media and 24-hour news cycles. The effects of a Black youth watching racially traumatic events (experiencing **vicarious racial trauma**) on TV or in their social media feed are almost inevitable. The impact of racial trauma on schooling is foreseeable, as well as its impact on grades, scores in standardized testing, and even school engagement. For example, according to the National Child Traumatic Stress Network (NCTSN, 2017), preschoolers who are exposed to vicarious racial insults or aggressions may exhibit behaviors in response to them. During classes, they may re-create a traumatic event, have difficulties with sleeping, struggle with low appetite, or react dramatically to incidents that are similar to what they were exposed to. These young students may not fully grasp media reports of racial trauma (such as a police shooting or beating) and may think each time an image is replayed on TV that it is actually happening again (NCTSN, 2017).

For school-aged children, the impact of racial trauma can also take a toll on their success in the classroom. For students in kindergarten through high school, they may have not only witnessed racially traumatic events, they may have also experienced discrimination, race-based stressors, and racist incidents firsthand. From an early age, Black students often experience or witness how differently Black people are treated in many areas of life. Unfortunately, racially traumatic experiences can even occur within their school. Schools that are predominantly Black are more likely to have onsite law enforcement and metal detectors than schools with largely white enrollment (Kidane & Rauscher, 2023). The daily routine of passing through metal detectors, removing clothing, emptying pockets, or even being wanded by security puts a strain on students and interferes with their learning (Levy, Heissel, Richeson, & Adam, 2016).

Levy and colleagues (2016) conducted a study that found psychological and biological responses to race-based social stress are pathways to disparities in educational outcomes. The study concluded that exposure to race-based stressors, such as the drive to outperform negative stereotypes, leads a student's body to produce more cortisol (a stress hormone). This heightened cortisol load is not common for the Black students' white peers. As a result, in the classroom, we may observe Black students who have more difficulty concentrating and less motivation (compared to their white peers), culminating in learning impairments.

School-based clinicians (guidance counselors, social workers, school psychologists) have the unique opportunity in their roles to provide teachers and administrators with professional development that highlights and acknowledges the achievement gaps between Black students and their white counterparts. Clinicians set the tone for the importance of creating a safe and learning-conducive environment for the school's Black students. Learn and understand the school's strengths and weaknesses (or potential areas of growth) in providing educational equity. A clinician assesses a school's strengths by examining areas where Black students are thriving and performing at par or above par. Areas of weakness are those where disparities exist in academic performance, discipline, or areas in which there are significant gaps between Black students and non-Black students. Outcomes are measured by operationalizing the problem and measuring areas of improvement. For example, a school's strength may be attendance; there are no significant differences between races in attendance. A school's weakness may be out-of-office referrals, with a disproportionate number of referrals for Black students based on the school's racial makeup or overall. The key is that the counselor draws on the school's strengths, addresses the areas where growth is needed, and measures the outcomes to determine the effectiveness of the intervention. Moreover, remember, change takes time!

In the case of Brian, who excels in some academic areas and struggles in others, the clinician can play a crucial role in his success. Notice which classes Brian thrives in and the strengths of the teachers in those classes. Do they know Brian on a personal level? Does the teacher invest time in Brian's strengths and areas of growth? Does the teacher truly "see" Brian for all he brings to class and not view him from a deficit model? Then the clinician can use their observation to assist the teachers who are struggling to educate Brian to his fullest potential. Not every teacher is the same and every teacher has their own methods of educating their students. However, is there a pattern in the classes where Brian struggles? For example, are all the Black males having issues? What are grades like across the entire class? How does the teacher connect to the Black-identified students in their class? Clinicians can bring their expertise into the room and a wealth of knowledge to Brian's situation.

School Discipline

While in English class, Tamarra, a Black female student, habitually tilts her chair back and drums on her desk with a pencil. One morning, she was engaging in this behavior while her teacher (a white female) was trying to teach the class. The teacher told Tamarra that she needed to stop, or she would be sent out of the classroom to the main office. Tamarra mumbled under her breath about the teacher and continued to drum but more quietly. The teacher, frustrated with this behavior, sent Tamarra to the office, with a slip claiming she had exhibited verbal disrespect.

Disrespectful. Defiant. Disruptive. Aggressive. Problem behavior. These descriptions are all based on subjective judgment, yet remain the frequent reasons Black children are threatened with being sent to the principal's office or ejected from the classroom. The difference in the ways in which a teacher may perceive a Black student's behavior versus that of a white student has been well documented (Alexander, Entwisle, & Thompson, 1987; Ferguson, 2003; Tenenbaum & Ruck, 2007; Tyson, 2002). In short, Black students are more likely than white ones to have their behavior in school described with such terms. The implication of this usage means Black students are more likely to spend less time in the classroom, become involved in the criminal justice system, and have fewer opportunities in the labor force (Zill & Wilcox, 2019; Monahan, VanDerhei, Bechtold, & Cauffman, 2014).

In a study by Wang and Del Toro (2021), school records, including discipline data, for a 3-year period were analyzed. Of the 2,381 sixth-, eighth-, and tenth-grade students from 12 schools in an urban Mid-Atlantic school district in the United States, 1,563 were white and 818 were Black. Wang and Del Toro found that over those 3 years, 26% of the Black students received at least one suspension for a minor infraction (dress code violation, use of cell phone in class, inappropriate language), compared with just 2% of white students. Several studies looking at the relationship among race, behavior, and suspension have not determined that Black students misbehave at higher rates than white students (Skiba, Chung, et al., 2014; Huang & Cornell, 2017; Skiba, Arredondo, & Williams, 2014; Skiba, Michael, Nardo, & Peterson, 2002; Skiba et al., 2011; Wallace, Goodkind, Wallace, & Bachman, 2008). Merely threatening to send a Black student to the main office can cause psychological damage as well as disrupt the engagement that student is experiencing in the classroom.

Interventions for excessive suspensions and out-of-classroom placements can come in many forms. One school district implemented a powerful group intervention created for students on the receiving end of such discipline. Students selected for the group were frequently removed from the classroom and sent to the office for misbehavior or had been suspended at least two times the prior year. These students had poor grades (failing two subjects or more during a single marking period) and poor school attendance. In addition to the group, the students were provided with individual counseling. The group was composed of eight boys. Although the weekly intervention required participating in group therapy, the importance of individual counseling cannot be understated—as the privacy of the individual sessions enabled students to confide in the facilitators and share personal concerns that they would not be likely to expose in a group setting. Many of the boys in these groups were referred for acting-out behavior, including fighting and other forms of aggression and violence in the school and community. The special connection each adolescent formed with his individual counselor was used in the group sessions to help resolve arguments or issues that developed between the group members. It is important to note that, in addition to violence prevention as a focus of the groups, the students often discussed other topics that were prominent in their lives, including relationships, their families, and dreams for the future.

In the case of Tamarra, it would have been important for the teacher to try and lay some groundwork between herself and Tamarra before the girl's behavior got so bad. A teacher and student having that kind of foundational relationship builds mutual respect. So if Tamarra was tapping her pencil and tilting her chair back and the teacher asked her to stop, she would have been more likely to stop because someone who cared about her and knew her had asked her to. With such prework, had something like this happened, the teacher could have ignored the behavior if it was not disrupting the class and discussed the incident with Tamarra at the next opportunity.

School-to-Prison Pipeline

Tyreek is a Black student in the 11th grade. After an incident with his teacher, he was arrested for assault by the police officer assigned to his school. The incident occurred when Tyreek returned to math class after a 3-day suspension for "repetitive verbal disrespect" in his math class. Upon his return to this class, Tyreek found himself further behind. He knew that if he failed the class, he would have to repeat it next year. His teacher (who is white) called on him several times to answer questions from the material he missed while suspended. Asked to solve another equation, Tyreek became frustrated and left the room, shouldering his teacher as she attempted to stop him from leaving by blocking the classroom door. The school police officer was called and Tyreek was placed in handcuffs; he was later arrested for assault on his teacher. The school district policy called for Tyreek to be expelled for this incident.

The United States has the highest incarceration rate in the world, and its prisons and jails are overwhelmingly filled with Black individuals. The pathways to prison for young Black individuals are many, but the starting point is often school. As noted earlier, many youth are on the receiving end of the racial trauma that occurs daily in schools, something which has lasting repercussions on their lives. Due to systemic and institutional racism, unconscious and conscious bias, Black students are targeted through discriminatory policies and procedures that mandate school suspension, expulsion, and arrest for an increasing array of minor student behaviors and rule infractions (Weissman, Cregor, Center, & Gainsborough, 2008).

When one thinks of racial trauma, the definition of trauma proposed by the *Diagnostic and Statistical Manual of Mental Disorders, Fifth Edition* (DSM-5) does not fit. Strictly following the DSM, one would say trauma is an event where a person must experience actual or threatened death, serious injury, or sexual violence. However, if we expand this definition to include harm that has long-term effects, then we can broaden it to include what is happening in schools across the country. That is, racial trauma has a significant impact on young Black students in the classroom that results in racial disparities in achievement, discipline, and graduation rates. All of these factors can lead to devastating results, including the school-to-prison pipeline.

According to the Prison Policy Initiative (Sawyer & Wagner, 2020), there are almost 2 million people in federal prisons, state prisons, local jails, juvenile correction facilities, immigration detention centers, and tribal jails across the United States. The system of mass incarceration disproportionately imprisons Black people, who are 12% of the U.S. population (according to the 2020 U.S. Census [Jones, Marks, Ramirez, & Rios-Vargas, 2021]) but 38% of the people in jails and prisons (Prison Policy Initiative, 2023). Our country has arrived at this juncture in numerous ways: policies that disproportionately target Black individuals, harsh policing in Black communities, and although the common saying is that "justice is blind," the justice system is, in fact, not blind. Let us take a closer look at how our young Black children enter the criminal justice system due to racial trauma in classrooms contributing to the school-to-prison pipeline.

The school-to-prison pipeline is defined as the policies and practices that directly and indirectly pushing students out of school and on a pathway to prison (American Civil Liberties Union, 2022). Black students face the trauma of being Black in school systems that are not built to support the varying unique needs of the Black student. Black students are more likely than others to be in the school-to-prison pipeline because they may start behind on social and academic skill due to limited enrichment from birth to age 5 (Nowicki, 2018). Black students may have poorer academic achievement and often have been held back at least one grade (Gregory, Skiba, & Noguera, 2010). They are more likely to be raised in a low-income single-parent household (McCarter, Venkitasubramanian, & Bradshaw, 2019). Finally, Black students have no or limited family history of postsecondary education (Assari, 2019).

Despite long-term declines in youth incarceration, the disparity between the rates at which Black and white youth are held in juvenile facilities has grown. For example, Sickmund and colleagues found that Black youth are more than four times as likely to be detained in juvenile facilities as their white peers (Sickmund, Sladky, Puzzanchera, & Kang, 2021). Additionally, 41% of youth in placement are Black, even though Black youth comprise only 15% of all youth across the United States (Puzzanchera, Sladky, & Kang, 2020). Race-based traumatic effects accumulate over time, having long-term impact on an individual's mental and physical health. Harsher discipline practices can cause long-lasting psychological, emotional, and even physical effects on Black students.

Schools with sworn police officers are more likely to criminalize normative adolescent behavior. Pushing and shoving are now considered "battery." Swiping headphones is now defined as "theft" or "robbery." Talking back is now regarded as "disorderly conduct." The list goes on. A chief judge of the juvenile court in Clayton County, Georgia, became an outspoken opponent of police in schools and the school-to-prison pipeline after observing that the presence of cops on school grounds resulted in 11 times as many students being sent to juvenile court (Nelson & Lind, 2015). He told Congress, "The prosecutor's attention was taken from the more difficult evidentiary and 'scary' cases—burglary, robberies, car thefts, aggravated assaults with weapons—to prosecuting kids that are not 'scary,' but made an adult mad!"

Black students are three times as likely to be arrested in schools as their white counterparts. In some states, Black girls are over eight times as likely to be arrested as white girls. A report by the ACLU, called *Cops and No Counselors* (Mann et al., 2019), analyzed data from the Civil Rights Data Collection and found that, in general, students of color are more likely to go to schools who have a police officer onsite, to be referred to law enforcement for their behaviors, and to be arrested at school. Black students make up 15.1% of school enrollment but almost 35% of students who are arrested in schools (Fisher & Devlin, 2024). This represents the worst disparity of any racial group. Additionally, according to the Office of Juvenile Justice and Delinquency Prevention (2022), Black youth are more likely to be referred to a juvenile court than white youth. Although many researchers have hypothesized on the reasons for this, the disparity remains (Leiber & Fix, 2019; Pope & Feyerherm, 1990; Pope, Lovell, & Hsia, 2002; Zane & Pupo, 2021).

The tangible consequences of being a Black student subjected to race-based traumatic stress are increased drop-out rates and risk of falling further behind in school. Using the case of Tyreek as an example, being arrested in his high school subjected him to exposure to possible trauma and abuse in a juvenile detention facility by staff or peers. He was separated from his family and community. Even more tragically, because he is 17 years old, the possibility exists that his case would have been transferred to adult court and he might have received extended incarceration. Tyreek walked out of the classroom and his teacher attempted to block his path, at which point he shouldered her to get past.

Multifaceted Framework for Interventions

Let us imagine four dissimilar racially trauma-informed scenarios in the case of Tyreek where things may have turned out differently.

Initial Suspension

Tyreek was suspended from school for 3 days for "repetitive verbal disrespect" toward his math teacher. Instead of suspension, what would it have looked like if the school clinician had conducted an intervention between the teacher and Tyreek, to assist the two in gaining a better understanding of each other? They could have learned what respect meant to each of them and what disrespect looked like as well. The doors of communication would have been opened, and Tyreek and his teacher could have worked on ways to better communicate in the classroom (see the discussion on mediation below). In this way, the clinician would have played a key role *before* suspension even occurred. Additionally, the clinician could have used the opportunity to coach the teacher in being culturally responsive.

There may have also been a reason behind Tyreek's behavior that his teacher is unaware of. He may be struggling in math class because he has a learning disability. Using data from the National Assessment of Educational Progress (NAEP), NCES, USDOE, and Institute of Education Sciences (IES), Morgan and colleagues (2019) found that Black students in the South are less likely to be identified as having learning disabilities when compared to their white peers. The role of a school clinician is to ensure there are criteria (such as having the school provide testing) to identify students with disabilities that are not just subjective and up to the referring teacher or parent. There is an overrepresentation of Black students in special education, however, and often these students are being referred for the wrong or inappropriate reasons (such as emotional disturbance). Quality trauma screenings can address whether acting-out behavior is related to trauma.

On the other hand, Tyreek may be bored in his math class because he is gifted, and the material being taught is not keeping his interest. Over the years, gifted programs have identified students who are white and Asian at notably higher rates than students who are identified as Black (USDOE, 2016; Worrell & Dixson, 2020; Yoon & Gentry, 2009).

Long et al. (2023) have indicated that nationally, among elementary schools with gifted education programs, Black students were only 55% as likely to be identified as gifted as white students.

Tyreek may also just be a young Black student who likes to speak up for himself! The clinician can take this opportunity to assist the teacher with discerning what is really going on with Tyreek. The clinician can also work with Tyreek on his tolerance of frustration and ways to handle situations like this that would not result in a physical altercation. For example, Tyreek could be coached to speak up for himself and articulate what he is experiencing and feeling in order to convey his message clearly to others. Additionally, the clinician can work with both the teacher and Tyreek on their communication in the classroom.

Returning from Suspension

According to the USDOE's OCR, Black students are nearly two times as likely as white students to be suspended without educational services (Smith et al., 2021). If we are not able to change the fact that Tyreek was suspended, let us look at how he was reacclimated back into school after being out for 3 days. He received no assistance in making up the work that he missed, or was even given make-up work. After his suspension, Tyree returned to class as if nothing had happened. However, by then he was 3 days behind his classmates—likely setting him up for further embarrassment and frustration.

Often, the school's hope is that the suspended student will have learned from the experience and thus make required behavioral changes. Yet, this is largely left up to chance. Reentry protocols are an attempt to make learning from a particular experience less random. During this process, a student is provided with increased structure as they again become accustomed to the demands of school. A good reentry program demonstrates collaboration and cooperation between adults (e.g., parents, teachers, administration) in the student's life and gives the student a way to make amends if necessary and feel welcomed back. This is a growing practice in the United States as restorative protocols become more prevalent in schools.

With Tyreek absent from school for several days, he has missed out on both the academic instruction that took place in his absence and school engagement. His peers are aware of what occurred in his math class. Tyreek's parents, teachers, and administrators are upset with or disappointed in him. Tyreek believes he has been mistreated, which comes with a host of feelings. After 3 days at home with disappointed parents, now he must face his teachers, administrators, and peers. Therefore, the goal of the reentry protocol is to assist Tyreek with efficiently returning to school and to set him up to succeed, socially and academically. The clinician guides Tyree in examining the initial problem that led to suspension, and then teaches or reteaches him the classroom and school expectations, and ultimately identifies necessary supports for him, and ensures those supports are put in place.

A clinician working in a school (or with a school) can spearhead a reentry program for all students who are suspended, if there is not one in place. This protocol will look different in every school; however, a few key elements should be present in any such program. First, it must involve the parents. Parental involvement can take on many different forms and should be racially trauma-informed, and allow the parent(s) to lead with how involved they are able to be. Some parents have the capacity to be very involved, while others do not. Parental involvement likely means taking a call from a counselor to discuss the reason for suspension, informing them of their rights and their child's. In this call, the counselor asks the parents about plans they have for their child while they are home, so the school can support them. As well, the counselor apprises parents of the school's reentry plan for when their child returns to school.

> COUNSELOR: Thank you for taking my call. Unfortunately, Tyreek was suspended today, and I would like to fill you in on what happened and what this means for Tyreek and his education. [The counselor then explains the circumstances that led to Tyreek's suspension.] I would like you to know that you and Tyreek have rights. Tyreek has the right to a due process appeal procedure for short-term suspensions. This is in the code of conduct and can be found online on our school's website. [The therapist informs Tyreek's parents of his rights and the school's process for appealing the suspension.]

PARENT: Thank you for letting us know. I don't think we'll appeal the suspension decision.

COUNSELOR: OK. Let's talk through how Tyreek can use his time while he is home on suspension. I can make sure his schoolwork gets sent home for the days that he will be out so he can do that while home. I know one of his favorite subjects is social studies, and I can ask the social studies teacher to send home an extra project that Tyreek might like to work on. [Here, the counselor mentions a school subject Tyreek enjoys, showing an investment in Tyreek's well-being.]

PARENT: Tyreek really likes basketball and sometimes goes to the YMCA to play. We can make arrangements for Tyreek to meet up with the coach during the suspension, so he can spend his time shooting hoops as well.

COUNSELOR: That sounds like a plan. I will be the reentry coordinator for Tyreek and you. My role is to coordinate Tyreek's assignments with administrators, his teachers, and any staff. I will be maintaining communication with you about the process and next steps. I will take care of all the referral paperwork and will collect data on how Tyreek does socially, emotionally, and academically after he returns. His reentry team will also consist of the vice principal, the teacher who suspended him, and his social studies teacher. [The reentry team should always have a counselor, an administrator, the teacher with whom the student has difficulty, and a trusted adult. In this case, the trusted adult is the social studies teacher.]

PARENT: This sounds like a good plan.

COUNSELOR: The day before Tyreek returns, I will invite you to the initial reintegration meeting with Tyreek. [Parent attendance ensures that the parents understand the intended outcomes: The student will be supported, relationships will be restored, etc.] I am also here to answer any questions you may have about the reintegration plan.

The second element in a school reentry program is counseling sessions (group or individual) for the student, tailored to the reason they were suspended. These sessions can take many forms. For example, they can take place during a nonessential class period. Some goals of these sessions include understanding the student's point of view of what happened and offering tips for ways to navigate similar situations in the future.

> COUNSELOR: Tyreek, thank you for meeting with me and explaining your point of view of the situation. I am glad you are open and willing to meet with your math teacher because it seems as though this is the only class where there are issues.
>
> TYREEK: Yeah, I don't know why she is always on my case, we just don't get along.
>
> COUNSELOR: This meeting with her will help clear up any miscommunications and hopefully help you to start fresh.
>
> TYREEK: OK, sounds good.
>
> COUNSELOR: Once we all meet together, we will identify ways for you to handle frustrating situations as well as assist your math teacher with managing her emotions and giving you an opportunity to excuse yourself when needed.

Finally, all reentry programs, especially for Black youth, should encompass building up the student's self-worth. The student can be reminded that they are not a "bad student," "defiant," or a "problem child" (or whatever label is being applied by others or the student themself). The clinician can also assist students with defining themselves and not allowing one incident to define them.

If all the student hears is "You're being a problem," or "This is why you're a problem," or "This is why you need to stop being a problem," the clinician risks the student tuning out and not listening to any of the conversation. Instead, start off the conversation by describing signs that the student's success is at risk and ask how you can support them.

Here is an example.

> "Thanks for coming down to talk to me. I know your goal is to pass your classes this year and I would like you to do so as well. However,

I am concerned. I noticed you were out of class due to 'disruptions' and then have not been completing assignments you missed. In addition, you have been doing poorly on tests and quizzes, which has caused your grades to go down. Is there something going on that I should know about so I can help you do better in this class?"

The clinician should relate every point they make back to the student's success. For instance, the student's behavior affects other students, which influences the student's learning environment, which then impacts the student. The clinician can also relay to the student that their behavior impacts the teacher, which affects the student's learning environment, which, in turn, impacts the student. Every student and every situation are different, but techniques like these reduce defensiveness and can strengthen the student's desire to do well in class.

Mediation

Mediation is an intervention in a dispute that aims to resolve it (Merriam-Webster, 2023). A high school in Brooklyn, New York, examined data showing which students were being disproportionately suspended. The school decided to empower students and teachers to solve disagreements through mediation sessions. These, in turn, created a strong sense of community within the school (WNYC, 2015). In the case of Tyreek, such a mediation intervention before his return to the classroom would have benefited both him and his teacher. Access to the mediation process may have given the teacher a chance to work with Tyreek sooner and staved off the incident that caused his arrest and expulsion from school.

The clinician could have walked the math teacher and Tyreek through any number of models of mediation before they encountered each other for the first time in the classroom where the shouldering incident occurred. For example, using an African-centered approach such as Hines and Sutton's Sankofa Violence Prevention Program utilizing facilitative mediation and transformative mediation models might have been beneficial (Hines et al., 2014). Sankofa Violence Prevention Program is a culturally sensitive, evidence-based, research-driven model for group treatment intervention originally designed for Black adolescents and other ethnic-minority youth. This violence prevention program is strength-based, highlighting the importance of resilience in high-risk situations. When African/Black-centered pedagogy is allowed to enter white spaces, the experience for Black students can be transformative. Facilitative mediation between Tyreek and his math teacher would allow examination of the conflict from each of their perspectives. The goal is to reach a resolution to the conflict that helps each of them to come together as a collective because in **African/Black psychology** the most important value is that the collective be the most salient element of existence. Another process the clinician can guide Tyreek and his math teacher through is transformative mediation. This is a much less structured approach that focuses on two key interpersonal processes: empowerment and recognition. The outcome is for both Tyreek and his teacher to feel supported by the clinician and each other as their conflict lessens and their relationship changes and strengthen.

Racially Competent Teaching

In her book *Raising Race Questions* (2015), Ali Michael of the Penn Center for the Study of Race and Equity in Education defines racially competent teaching as "the skills and attitudes required to develop and maintain healthy cross-racial relationships, notice and analyze racial dynamics, and confront racism in the environment and in oneself" (p. 9). Earlier in the chapter, we discussed the shortcomings of teacher preparation programs. The solutions start with the teacher's educational programs' recognizing that racial competency is not a skill one is born with. Racial competency involves a continuous learning process, revisited on a regular basis.

In the case of Tyreek, a 17-year-old Black adolescent, many things are happening for him developmentally at the same time: He is forming his racial identity, understanding his gender identity, navigating his relationships with his peers, thinking about his future, and more. Having a teacher call on him, in front of his peers, for answers to questions he was not in school to learn was embarrassing. His ego and pride were hurt; he felt humiliated. In this situation, the school clinician could have assisted his math teacher with literature, trainings, and resources to help equip her with the skills to teach Black (adolescent) students in a racially trauma-informed way. This could have been accomplished through schoolwide professional development with the staff that focused on relationship building and trauma-informed classroom practices. In addition to professional development, the clinician could have built a relationship with Tyreek's teacher so that she would have felt comfortable coming to the clinician for help.

Once again, these four kinds of intervention are examples of ways in which to intervene in a trauma-informed way with a student like Tyreek. These interventions require a team approach, collaboration, and sensitivity to the lived experience of the youth. The outcomes and takeaways from these approaches for youth, parents, teachers, administrators, and counselors can and will be powerful.

CHAPTER TAKEAWAYS

One of the major goals of a school clinician is to foster emotionally healthy children. That goal applies to all children. However, for Black children, clinicians need to be intentional about identifying and addressing the behavioral nuances that arise from how kids make sense of and cope with the racial trauma they are exposed to in their lives. Intentionality includes:

- Knowing who is teaching the Black child. Do teachers need coaching, support, and education about how to reach the child? This is an opportunity for clinicians to use their position of influence in schools to call out aspects of the educational experiences that are not conducive to their well-being and may be perpetuating racial stereotypes and discrimination.

- Identifying any systemic issues in the school environment that disproportionately affect the achievement of Black students. By doing this, clinicians can eliminate the many excuses as to why Black student achievement is not on par with or higher than that of their white counterparts.

- Drawing on and highlighting the strengths of the teachers who are getting it right. Emphasize the areas where teachers need more growth and offer the tools they need to be successful in the classroom. Professional development can be a transformative experience for the teacher, and their students will benefit. Understand and address the impact of disproportionate and harsh discipline on Black students. As a clinician, you have a unique position in the student's life and within the system in which they are learning. Remember to leverage your knowledge with school administration to guide them to regularly review discipline policies and procedures. Collect the data. Identify for administrators the aspects of policies that disproportionately harm Black students. Additionally, work with teachers on classroom management skills aimed to support the most vulnerable children.

CHAPTER 6

Black and Blue
Working with Law Enforcement

> I can't breathe.
> —Eric Garner[1]

"I can't breathe," "Hands up, don't shoot," and Silence

In July 2014, on every newsstand and in every news outlet, the images were unavoidable: a Black man in a chokehold lying on a New York City street uttering the words "I can't breathe" until he lost consciousness. Eric Garner, 44, was allegedly selling untaxed loose cigarettes when local police officers approached him. This encounter ultimately cost Garner his life. During that same summer, across the country, images of an 18-year-old Black male, Michael Brown, lying dead on the street after an encounter with a white officer, Darren Wilson, in Ferguson, Missouri, also permeated our TV screens.

For months, the media and many people's everyday conversations included discussions of the two cases. Chants of "I can't breathe" were heard across the country, and images of young Black men with their hands in the air, often with the caption "Hands up, don't shoot,"

---

[1] Eric Garner was a Black man, killed in New York City by an NYPD officer who put him in a prohibited chokehold while arresting him. Video footage of the incident generated widespread national attention and raised questions about the use of force by law enforcement.

appeared all over the Internet, at demonstrations and protests. On November 24, 2014, a St. Louis County grand jury decided not to indict Officer Wilson, finding that he had shot Michael Brown in self-defense. About a week later, on December 4th, the Richmond County grand jury in New York decided not to indict Daniel Pantaleo, the policeman seen on video putting Eric Garner in a chokehold. Hundreds of demonstrations nationwide sprung up in response to these two cases, as well as countless demonstrations against police brutality.

Clinicians working with law enforcement and within law enforcement settings are in a unique position to examine the impact of racial trauma from two perspectives. The first perspective is that of individuals with careers in law enforcement, and the second is that of the policing and criminal justice system itself, which was founded on systemic and institutionalized racism. In their profession, police officers have a high probability of experiencing trauma, which can then be compounded when they face racially traumatic events involving one of their own. Additionally, Black-identified officers may experience significant symptoms of trauma triggered by national racialized events in addition to their own personal experiences with racism.

Witnessing the disparate treatment of Black and white individuals by police officers can be unsettling for many. For Black individuals, both civilians and those in law enforcement, knowing the history of policing in America alone can increase the likelihood of trauma responses when interacting with police, or when hearing about negative police-related incidents. This chapter explores the psychological impact of such police-related racially traumatic events on law enforcement agencies and offers clinical guidance for supporting those working in law enforcement.

When we speak about racial trauma and policing, we often think about officers abusing Black individuals, and the impact that has on the Black community. However, it is important also to understand the psychological impact racial trauma (particularly police-related racial trauma) has on Black individuals who wear the uniform.

Among NYC probation and corrections officers, one would think incidents such as those described above would be hot topics of conversation. However, working with these departments in 2014, one of us (J. R. J.-D.) found that silence reigned among the officers. Men and women in uniform frequently did not have the words to begin or sustain a conversation about racial trauma related to policing in America. So many of these officers walked on eggshells at work. Individuals were afraid of saying something wrong, afraid of offending someone, and many thought, "We don't have these conversations here at work."

This silence at the time stemmed from police officers' difficulty articulating their experience of vicarious racial trauma, which refers to the reaction a person has when seeing or hearing about a traumatizing racial incident happening to someone else. For many officers, it is difficult to reconcile that there are systemic racial issues in law enforcement and that they are, by choice, part of this same system. Such individuals do not identify themselves as the "problem"; they see themselves as doing their job the best they can in a flawed system. In addition, this difficulty may be compounded in officers who identify as Black.

Officers (patrol, corrections, probation, and others) experience high rates of trauma while performing their duties (Myles, 2020). Each day, they may face being assaulted, becoming involved in shootings, responding to suicides or homicides, or observing a violent assault or fight. Unsurprisingly, this trauma often goes unaddressed, which, as stated earlier, can lead to **burnout**, turnover, or even posttraumatic stress disorder (PTSD; Myles, 2020). Significant symptoms can be activated by direct or indirect exposure to racially traumatic events that occur on the job or are reported in the media.

People expect officers to perform at their highest potential and make the right decisions under extreme stress. Officers are not only supposed to be healthy physically and mentally, but they must also maintain high performance levels in the line of duty. Officers are expected to be stronger and more courageous than "ordinary people." While living up to these standards can lead to promotions, praise, and accolades, the pressure and stress of doing that can also lead to poor psychological well-being. Moreover, working in a culture where such high expectations are normalized makes it difficult for officers to ask for psychological help when needed.

Each officer has their own background and identity outside of being an officer, their own personal thoughts and feelings. At the end of their day, they return home and to their community and assume the role of a parent, spouse, sibling, friend, and so on. When highly publicized racially traumatic events occur involving law enforcement, the impact on Black police officers is no less hard than on the average Black individual in the community.

The difference is that often there is not a space for an individual in uniform to openly express the impact racial trauma has on their lives. Among their colleagues, an "us versus them" mentality is pervasive, often forcing individuals in uniform to feel obligated to pick a side in societal debates about racism, civil rights, and discrimination. At times, that mentalitycan impede officers from seeking psychological help.

Working with Individual Officers after Police-Racialized Trauma

Kim Thompson is a 33-year-old Black officer. She entered individual therapy with a white therapist and presented with anxiety and panic attacks. Her symptoms began after she had heard about the shooting of an 11-year-old Black boy in Mississippi. The child had called the police for help and, upon arrival, an officer shot him. Kim also has an 11-year-old Black son, and hearing about the shooting heightened her fear for his safety. This fear became excessive and problematic in her life. She and her therapist scheduled 10 sessions of cognitive-behavioral therapy (CBT)—Kim kept only 5 of them. Kim showed no improvement on objective measures and reported no change. Her Beck Anxiety Inventory (BAI; Beck, Epstein, Brown, & Steer, 1988) scores remained markedly high (indicating no reduction in symptomatology), she continued to significantly reduce her son's activities outside of the house, and she started missing work for fear of his whereabouts after school. Nevertheless, Kim continues to minimize the impact that the vicarious racial trauma is having on her everyday life. She refuses any suggestions for making changes, such as limiting her news intake related to the killings of young Black boys, and practicing self-care by engaging in activities that she enjoys and that make her happy. She also told her therapist she misses so many sessions because she is fearful someone will find out she is in therapy. Each time the therapist attempts to point out the lack of Kim's progress, Kim responds with comments like "It's a hopeless situation and that's that" and "What's the point of doing anything different? Someone can just come and shoot my son and take the only thing worth living for away from me." She also laments that she is not getting anything out of this therapy. The therapist begins to find working with Kim to be tiresome, repetitive, and frustrating, and must struggle to manage their own reactions to Kim's responses.

Officers can be seen as a resistant population when seeking mental health treatment. Mental illness is often stigmatized in the Black community, and this is particularly so among the ranks in law enforcement. Officers frequently believe addressing their mental health will impede their ability to move up the career ladder and possibly lead to their being labeled as unfit for the job. Introducing **motivational interviewing (MI)**, a therapeutic interview delivery style, can help in providing care with treatment-resistant populations such as police officers (Hohman, 2021). MI involves enhancing a person's motivation to change by understanding their own motivations, listening with empathy, and empowering them to move toward their goals. Using MI with officers can encourage them to become an active participant in their change process by evoking their intrinsic motivations for change.

In the case of Kim, MI could have made a difference in her engagement in therapy and her work toward her goals. The therapist could have tapped into what her motivations were to help Kim change her behavior. Kim called to schedule therapy for a reason. The therapist can start there, with Kim's desire to change. In cross-racial therapy with Kim, the therapist should listen with empathy about Kim's fears for her child.

Validation is an important step in MI. It is not just about recognizing emotions, but about creating a judgment-free zone where the client's emotions are accepted. By using different forms of validation, a therapist can build a stronger connection with their clients while creating an environment that promotes healing. In the case of Kim, the therapist would validate Kim's fears and recognize that these fears are real threats in the world toward her child. Saying things like "It's understandable that you feel that way," "Most people would feel the same in your situation," and "You have every right to feel afraid," the therapist can use MI-inspired prompts to get Kim to explore her wants and needs in the session. This is an opportunity for Kim to explore how she wants to live her life and how she wants her son to live his.

> James Jackson is a 54-year-old Black corrections officer working at a large correctional facility in the young adult building (ages 18–21). He has worked at this jail for almost 25 years. He presented to therapy with difficulty sleeping, using alcohol to assist with his insomnia, and getting into frequent arguments with his wife. According to him, he was only at the clinic because his wife encouraged him to seek counseling.

During sessions, James and the therapist spoke about his sleeping patterns and his stressors, and they found ways to build his coping skills to ease his stressors. At that time, the term "racial trauma" was not at the forefront of many therapists' minds. As their sessions unfolded, themes of race, harassment, and identity began to surface. Officer Jackson entered therapy a few weeks after Philando Castile, a 32-year-old Black man, had been fatally shot during a traffic stop by a police officer in Minneapolis. Castile was licensed to carry a weapon and informed the officer that he had the gun in his possession. The officer told Castile not to reach for it, and Castile repeatedly stated that he was not reaching for the gun. However, the officer proceeded to fire seven close-range shots at Castile, hitting him five times. Castile died about 20 minutes after being shot.

This incident was live-streamed on a popular social media platform by Castile's girlfriend who was with him at the scene, and it almost instantly gained international attention—including the attention of Officer Jackson. Within a few weeks, he could not sleep, began drinking more, and directed all his frustrations toward his wife. He mentioned in passing during one of his sessions how disappointed he was that the country could just move past the killing of Philando Castile, on to the next thing. He took a deep breath, looked at the therapist, and said, "I may be an officer at work, but out there I'm just another ni***r everyone sees as a threat." He spoke about how many times he was stopped by his fellow officers while driving, and pointed out that if he had not had his badge on him, he did not know what might have happened. While speaking with his therapist, he conveyed his frustration, anger, and sadness. He raised his voice as he became emotional and even teared up at times. The public slayings of the last few years (Trayvon Martin, Tamir Rice, Michael Brown, Eric Garner, George Floyd, and Philando Castile whose story initially activated him) had continued to pile up in his psyche, and he was holding onto a lifetime of unjust treatment, leading to anger, resentment, frustration, and grief that he had no way of processing or gaining mastery over.

At this time, the therapist simply let Officer Jackson vent and emote. However, if Officer Jackson had been given a space where he was validated and his feelings were normalized, he might have had an opportunity to see the impact that vicarious racial trauma had had on him. Had the therapist had the tools, as outlined below, they would have been able to assist Officer Jackson in healing from the racial trauma he experienced, rather than listening to him vent about it.

Techniques for Working with Black Officers

Addressing racial trauma is different from coping with racial trauma. For example, imagine it is cold in the room you are in as you are reading this book. How do you cope with the cold? You decide to put on a sweater. Putting on a sweater helps you deal with the cold room, but it does not change the fact that the room is cold. Imagine after you put on the sweater, you then get up and change the temperature in the room. Now you have addressed the problem and can stop coping and take off your sweater. While clinicians should not shoulder the burden of feeling as if it's their sole responsibility to eradicate the systems that promote race-based trauma, clinicians can ensure their therapy rooms—where we have control—is where we will give space for people to explore and find healing and support strategies.

We do not want our clients to just cope with racial trauma; we want to address the impact it is having on their lives. Clients are coping with racial trauma in many different ways. For example, they may not watch the news any more. They may become numb to the stories of Black individuals being hurt, harmed, or killed because of the color of their skin. They may even become hyper-vigilant, avoiding anything and everything that remind them of the trauma. Officer Jackson's form of coping was using alcohol to numb the pain as well as putting up "armor" that kept people at a distance, including his wife. There are a number of therapeutic techniques a therapist can use while treating or consulting with clients who work in law enforcement that go beyond teaching coping skills.

Being Seen, Heard, and Understood

The role of a clinician is to truly see their client, beyond what the client is presenting. This is not an easy feat, and with Black clients, it requires a particular sensitivity and skill. From early in their lives, Black clients endure a barrage of unwelcomed and unjustified negative stereotypes and messages from the world around them. The client may have internalized many of these messages. This internalization places the person behind these messages, such that who they really are remains unseen. What the clinician sees is an anxious and depressed client, a client who drinks too much, a client burned out for having to be twice as good in this world to have half the chance as their white counterparts, a person struggling with anxiety, and even who perhaps wants to die.

For the clinician to properly treat their client, they need to see them—and that means they need to really hear their client's story. The therapist can assist the client with painting a whole picture of what is affecting their lives. Consider Officer Jackson, presenting with marital concerns, heavy drinking, and built-up frustration and anger. These concerns are just the outward manifestation of internalized devaluation (Hardy, 2013). As Ken Hardy stated, "Internalized devaluation is a direct by-product of racism, inextricably linked to the deification of whiteness and the demonization of non-white hues" (2013, p. 25). Behind the badge, Officer Jackson is a Black man who is devalued in this society because he is Black. The therapist needed to create a space where Officer Jackson felt seen and valued. This was done by acknowledging all of who Officer Jackson was and allowing him to bring his whole self to the space. He was finally able to speak about the impact the killing of a Black man by police had on him. Officer Jackson grappled with the fact that he was both a Black man and an officer.

Normalizing Clients' Reactions

In the wake of racially traumatic events, Black officers often find themselves struggling to reconcile their dual identities, that of an officer and that of a Black person in America. When conversations of police-related racial trauma emerge, it may be hard for a Black officer to "pick a side." If a Black officer identifies with and speaks up for a Black victim, then they are betraying their colleagues in Blue. If they identify with and speak up for an officer involved in an incident, then they are betraying their Black community. This duality is an unavoidable phenomenon. The "normal reaction" is, instead, the no–win dilemma the officer feels, and the pain of having divided loyalties, and the stress of carrying around (and having to answer for) these two identities.

Fear, anxiety, worry about personal safety, anger, sadness, grief, shame, helplessness, diminished self-worth, numbness, shock, and disbelief: These are all normal reactions to horrific racially traumatic events that occur in the world and to the Black clients we serve. Let your clients know this. Reinforce that each person processes emotions at their own pace; there are no time limits on emotions, especially those that are the result of interpersonal racial trauma.

Monitoring for Signs of Stress and Vicarious Trauma

Walter Howard Smith, Jr. (2010) described the impact of racial trauma on African Americans. He noted six different symptoms that can show up, all of which are germane to working with Black police officers:

1. **Increased vigilance and suspicion:** Individuals facing chronic racial trauma may become suspicious of social institutions (schools, agencies, government). This can show up as avoiding eye contact with others, or only trusting people within their social and family relationships. A good example of increased vigilance in the Black community emerged with respect to vaccines during the COVID-19 pandemic. Many Black individuals refused to be vaccinated because they did not trust the government or the medical community. Historically, the government and the medical community harmed the Black community purposely in

the areas of experimentation without knowledge, such as the infamous Tuskegee experiments (Bates & Harris, 2004), and even sterilization of Black women (Stern, 2020). These historical, racially driven outrages became traumatizing for many Black people. When the government decided to offer free COVID vaccines, many in the community were suspicious of them and declined treatment.

2. **Increased sensitivity to threat:** Navigating a majority-white society as a Black person can feel like living on the balls of your feet, ever ready to pounce or fight. The individual has a defensive posture and a heightened sensitivity to being disrespected and shamed. This sensitivity develops over time because racially traumatic events do not occur once; they keep occurring. These recurring events, and the chronic stress they provoke, may leave a Black person feeling the need to stay on guard to avoid being harmed either physically or psychologically. Moreover, this heightened sensitivity can appear in the form of individuals' avoiding places and situations, and even not taking low-level risks.

3. **Increased psychological and physiological symptoms:** Unresolved racial traumas increase chronic stress. This, in turn, leads to increased risks for depression and anxiety disorders. Clients may present to a therapist with "depression" or "anxiety" that has intruded on their lives, to the point where family and social relationships are being affected. Clinicians should look beyond the typical diagnosis and strive to find what is driving these disorders.

4. **Increased alcohol and drug usage:** Exposure to racial trauma does not automatically lead to use (or abuse) of drugs and alcohol. Yet, the stress of living with their irreconcilable roles (professional vs. personal) can leave Black police officers feeling as if they must cope with racially traumatic events on their own. How do they cope? Perhaps it's by drinking a glass of wine to help them fall asleep. One glass today turns into two glasses tomorrow night, and so on. In time, the person finds they cannot even get to sleep without the use of substances. This kind of coping technique can be adaptive, but when substances are continuously used and the underlying problem is not addressed, the adaptive coping skill becomes maladaptive.

5. **Narrowed sense of time:** Individuals living in a prolonged state

of real or perceived danger because of their identity do not develop a sense of future. While working with young Black adults at the Rikers Island detention center in NYC, a clinician would often talk to them about their future when they got out of jail. One young person replied, "Miss, I don't have a future. I'll probably be dead and end up on someone's T-shirt." These youth were contending with community violence and a host of systemic issues, yet embedded in all of their stories was their identity: They were young Black males in a society that does not value young Black male lives. When dealing with a narrowed sense of time, Black individuals do not set long-term goals and can view dying as an expected near-term outcome.

6. **Increased aggression:** Increased aggression can take on many forms. In the case of Officer Jackson, he initiated verbal arguments with his wife. This was one of the reasons he sought therapy. The clinician should look for areas of the client's life where there is discord. Do interpersonal problems exist with individuals who would typically be a part of their support system? Is there an on-the-job conflict that seems disproportionate to the situation presented? Is the client taking out anger on their loved ones?

As a clinician, think of how you would cope with the threat of being hurt, harmed, or killed because of the way you look? Would you become defiant? Try to appear tough and impenetrable? Understand that a common way of coping with racial trauma is to attempt to control one's physical and social environment. To the world, this may look like aggressive behavior.

Monitoring signs and symptoms is a key step in recognizing the impact of racial trauma. Clients may not be clear when they come in for treatment that they are suffering from a racially traumatic event (or from chronic consistent microaggressions, **macroassaults,** profiling, and fear of being hurt, harmed, or killed because of their identity). Examining such symptoms can point to the problem. Symptoms give us clues as to where to take a closer look. They offer clues to further explore and may signal a need to investigate possible exposure to racial trauma or race-based stressors. Once the root of the problem is determined, then, and only then, can it be adequately addressed.

Working with Law Enforcement Agencies after Racialized Trauma

> A county probation department was having trouble with communication and morale after a series of racially charged events at the local and national levels. A few officers of color began displaying "Black Lives Matter" at the bottom of their emails. Two officers hung "Blue Lives Matter" flags in their offices. When conversations about the events happening in the country took place, that dialogue would become heated between some officers, while others hung back and said nothing. Eventually, the chief of the department made the decision that no one could reference or display either Black Lives Matter or Blue Lives Matter items or slogans. Additionally, all conversations on racial incidents were essentially shut down from being discussed at work. The therapist then received an email from the training office inquiring about introducing racial trauma training to their entire department.

Department Culture

Clinical training programs may ask clinicians to visualize themselves sitting in offices meeting individually with clients, conducting counseling with families, or facilitating groups. There is a whole other role for a clinician, that of a consultant. This clinician consultant can have a massive impact on organization or in a community by consulting with various agencies, in this case law enforcement agencies. The clinician can assist with changing dangerous practices that may lead to racial trauma.

When working with a team or an entire department, the first step of engagement is understanding the culture of the law enforcement agency you are working with. To do this, begin by listening to their stories. A great question to start with is "What prompted you to *want to* bring a racial trauma training to your department?" It is easy to go into a meeting with a training program already created and a contract in hand, offering the same workshop to this new department that you offered to the last one. The result of such a canned intervention is often initially helpful discussions, but no lasting impact. Why? Teaching information helps a person gain knowledge, but it does not take the additional step of demonstrating how to *apply* the knowledge and skills in the context of the culture of their department. For example, in a law enforcement department that has a culture where it is difficult to talk about race as it relates to implicit bias on the job, it would be important to focus on educating how implicit bias shows up specifically in the department. This specificity allows participants to see how these terms manifest themselves in real life as it relates to their job.

In this case, the consultant worked in a department that was unsure of how to navigate differences of opinions. On the one hand, there were officers who supported the **Black Lives Matter (BLM)** movement and were deeply impacted by seeing Black individuals harmed, or even killed, at the hands of police. These individuals understood that even though they were law enforcement, they were Black people first. On the other hand, there was the **Blue Lives Matter** movement supporters who deeply identified as being law enforcement. They believed that officers were blamed for everything wrong with the justice system, and because of the hatred toward officers, many were fearful of being in uniform while on duty. Both sides felt deeply committed and rooted to either the Black Lives Matter movement or the Blue Lives Matter movement. Additionally, both groups were deeply offended by the other group's chosen affiliation and use of these terms. Each side was hoping for the department to decide which group was right. Instead, the department shut down the conversation and told both groups they were no longer allowed to express such views in the office.

This kind of scenario, with departmental splits and interpersonal tension, is not uncommon in law enforcement offices. Working with departments that are split on opposite sides of a particular racial event is difficult territory to navigate. As trained clinicians, we are not taught how to work in such contexts. Clinicians do not hold all the answers and, in fact, should approach the department in a way that emphasizes this. For instance, if a clinician went into training with this agency and told the Black Lives Matter group that they had the right perspective and laid out all the evidence and all the information supporting this movement, that clinician would lose the attention and credibility of the rest of the officers. If a clinician instead claimed the Blue Lives Matter movement was valid and offered all the evidence to show why this movement was important, the clinician would likewise lose all credibility. The goal in an intervention like this is not to decide who is right, but to get everyone to have a respectful discussion.

When working with departments amid local or national racial trauma, the key is to bring everyone to the table. This requires understanding departmental culture and not alienating any one group. The ultimate goal is to have everyone understand racial trauma and that it has a real impact on the individuals and the system in which they are embedded. Coming to the table does not mean agreeing on a topic. It certainly does not entail convincing the person across from them who is right and who is wrong. Rather, getting the parties to come to the table requires creating a situation in which department staff are willing to speak their truth and listen to others' truths, which will be different from their own. A shift in department culture takes time; however, planting the seeds of mutual understanding can go a long way.

Fostering and (Re)building Relationships

After the first step, understanding the department culture and prompting everyone in the department to view different perspectives, is completed, the next step would be to find strengths to draw on. It all starts with the relationship. When conducting a group-facilitated training, remind participants that they may spend more time with each other than they do at home with their families. Tell them the work they do is hard and sometimes never-ending. Remind them that they have been there for each other when their children graduated, when a spouse or partner died, when someone received a promotion, and many other major life events. The reason a clinician starts with the relationship is this: There should be a clear understanding that those around the table are not strangers. They are colleagues who work together every day; these colleagues most likely do not have malice or malcontent in their heart, or a desire to harm each other. The foundation of addressing racial trauma in police departments means starting with the relationship of those who make up the department.

Voluntary or Mandatory?

The department needs to decide whether the interventions triggered by racial trauma should be mandatory or voluntary. When training is mandatory, some people may attend begrudgingly, feeling as if it is just another hoop they must jump through or a box they must check. When training is voluntary, the same few people who want to learn and grow tend to show up, and, typically, the most marginalized individuals who are most deeply affected by racial trauma are those present. In addition to these individuals, there is inevitably a sprinkling of white-identified participants who want to support their marginalized peers. For more impactful change, clinicians should encourage their organizational client to require mandatory training and conversations. After the foundational principles have been taught and relationships built, then departments can make future discussions and participation about race in learning spaces voluntary. However, even with the learning spaces being voluntary, everyone in the department should pick a space in which to participate. Because participating in a conversation is mandatory, giving some voice and choice to the participants even in the smallest ways, for instance, which meeting they can join, is impactful.

For the probation department in the example above, the therapist spent a year conducting 3-hour mandatory training sessions with all the officers. Make sure that everyone on the payroll is being trained. Include officers, administration, and leadership in the organization, not just a frontline staff. Most police, corrections, and probation departments are large. Therefore, these trainings were delivered to groups of no more than 20 to 25 people per session. The reason for smaller group sizes is that in a mass group training many people do not pay attention and have the opportunity to speak up and ask questions.

Also, consider the makeup of the small groups. There are pros and cons to having supervisors and managers in the same groups with the frontline staff. One way to break up the training is to separate all the frontline officers into small groups where they receive the racial trauma training together. Supervisors and managers move to a separate training session. The benefit of this approach is that it allows each group an opportunity to speak freely without fear of retaliation or looking bad in front of each other. Sometimes speaking among one's peers is more comfortable than speaking around supervisors or supervisees. A drawback is that separation by rank can also create an "us and them" hierarchy. Additionally, neither group will know how the other feels about racial situations. However, it is usually better to keep all ranks together and establish the foundation for creating a "brave space."

A brave space is different from a safe space. A facilitator cannot create a "safe space" for everyone present in the training. Safety means something different to everyone attending, and the facilitator is unable to meet the safety needs of everyone. Therefore, the goal is to create a space where individuals can be brave and speak what is on their mind, knowing that others may be supportive, unsupportive, positive, or even judgmental regarding what is said.

Trainings

As the first step in training, the clinician helps the group understand *why* it is valuable to learn about racial trauma and *why* it is important to have these difficult conversations. If the training is mandatory, many people attending it will want to tune out. As previously noted, the facilitator's role is to find a way to bring these individuals to the table. This is done by validating the group's experiences. This does not mean dumbing down, watering down, or making racial trauma easier to swallow. It means helping individuals less personally affected by racial trauma to find an emotional connection to people who are most impacted by racial trauma, and giving examples that allow people to stand in each other's shoes.

Here is an exercise a clinical trainer could use to instill a sense of common ground:

> "Imagine before this training I came in and told you that down the block an accountant was shot and killed while doing taxes. You might be shocked that something happened so close to where we are. You may be sad for the accountant's family. We would continue with our training. You would remember the story a few days from now. But maybe within a few weeks, it will fade from your memory. Now imagine I came in here and told you an officer was just shot and killed while on duty right down the block. That news would hit you differently. You might think, 'That could have been me.' Or, 'That could have been my partner.' Or, 'That could have been any one of us in this room.' We most likely would cancel the day's training. You would remember this for a while to come."

The clinician can go on to say that this is what racial trauma is like. When you see someone hurt, harmed, or killed because of the way they look or their identity, and they look and identify just like you, the harm is felt differently. We are all impacted differently based on our identities.

The second step during a training is to create a common language. Often the reason why individuals have difficulty discussing race is because people define relevant terms differently. For example, someone calls a particular situation a "racist act," another calls the same situation an "act of discrimination," and yet another calls this situation a "microaggression." If the individuals do not know how each person is defining the situation, misunderstandings can occur. The clinician should spend some time going over the definitions of some of the most frequently used terms when talking about racial trauma. Once a common language is created, there will be fewer misunderstandings about the terms that individuals use to describe their experiences.

The third step is allowing time for discussion of the impact various racially traumatic events have had on the individuals in training. Breaking up into smaller groups of four or five during a session allows for a more intimate setting, one where individuals can speak freely. For example, during a training, a Black officer shared a racially biased incident that occurred during lunch with his colleagues. He walked into the lunchroom with a red drink in hand, and a colleague said aloud to everyone in the room, "Of course, YOU would be drinking Kool-Aid!" There is a common stereotype that Black people always drink Kool-Aid. The Black officer was the butt end of a racial joke, and he became embarrassed in front of his peers. The impact was that he stopped consuming red-colored drinks in the lunchroom and remained fearful of being singled out again. When the training group reconvened, he shared with all the impact that this incident had had on him. This humanized the concepts at play and the impact racialized events have on real people. The whole group was thus able to hear and give feedback to what others were saying in real time.

Again, the entirety of the training itself should be tailored to the department. However, core subjects may include addressing why the topic of racial trauma matters for officers; acknowledging that the work officers do leads to direct exposure to trauma, making the exposure to racial trauma a compounding event; describing the impact racial trauma has on the individual and systems; and proposing techniques to address racialized events as an individual and as a department.

Next Steps

After training everyone, it is necessary to offer tangible next steps. A consultant or trainer will have only limited time with the department. It would be a shame if discussions stopped after the training ended. Having a separate meeting with individuals who hold power within the organization gives a clearer picture of the commitment these individuals have toward changing their departments, and creating environments that allow people to express their true feelings around race and racial trauma in constructive ways. In the example above, after the intervention, the chief of the department wanted an open dialogue between individual officers and no longer felt the need to shut down conversations. The next step was to then train the supervisors on how to facilitate such conversations with their supervisees. Going through tips and techniques that are all evidence-based on how to facilitate conversations based on race is crucial. One tip to give individuals to assist in facilitating discussions about race is to offer them example language, such as:

> "I've been thinking about you lately: everything that has been going on and the racial trauma you might be experiencing. Would you like to talk about anything?"

> "We don't usually talk about race at work, but I've been wondering how the news has been impacting you lately."

> FOR WHITE OFFICERS
> "I know that I am white and not of your race, and can't possibly understand what you might be going through. I want you to know that I am open to hearing anything you need to say right now."

> "I can't begin to understand what this must be like for you."

Another tip is not personalizing a person's response or anger to a racialized event. Also, try not to become defensive when being **called out**. Calling out someone means letting a person know that they are being offensive and disrespectful in the moment in front of the individuals who were present when the incident occurred. This allows more people to hold the person accountable. Finally, use **calling in**, a practice whereby a person is spoken to in private about a racial transgression and the impact this had on the person confronting them and possibly others who were present.

Just providing handouts or discussion points, and telling the supervisors to lead such conversations when they have never done so before, is setting them up for failure. Allow space and time for them to ask questions to really delve into the material and to set a tone for the department; also reassure them that they do not have to have all the answers to hold open the space for these kinds of conversations. One of the biggest fears of supervisors is "What if things go wrong and people start arguing and disagreeing about a topic?" Let them know that this is not uncommon and advise them that they should always bring the conversation back to the *relationship*, making it clear that although someone's intent was not to cause hurt or harm, their comments or behavior can still hurt.

CHAPTER TAKEAWAYS

- Whether working with Black individuals in law enforcement or working with entire law enforcement agencies, it is important to acknowledge the psychological impact of police-related racial trauma. Law enforcement can be seen as a resistant population so knowing which techniques work best will be key.

- When bringing racially traumatic events forward in therapy, ensure that your client is seen and heard. Normalize the reactions of the individual and the systemic reaction of the agency. Racially traumatic events at the hands of law enforcement can make folks feel as if they need to pick a side of the fence to land on.

- Remind the individuals in the system that the issue is not about picking a side; rather, the focus should be on the impact the events had on them and the people around them. Finally, yet importantly, assist with monitoring signs of racial traumatic stress.

- The symptoms outlined in this chapter (anxiety and panic attacks, difficulty sleeping, using alcohol to assist with insomnia, getting into frequent arguments) are not specific to someone experiencing a racial trauma. Therefore, it is important to understand what lies beneath and why the person is experiencing these symptoms. Remember, tracing back to the origin of the symptoms to the root cause of the problem is a clear way to identify the problem and address its impact.

CHAPTER 7

The Talk
Helping Parents and Children with Racial Trauma

> The Black family of the future will foster our liberation, enhance our self-esteem, and shape our ideas and goals.
> —Dorothy Height, an African American civil rights leader and women's rights activist

Edward is a 14-year-old African American male you are meeting for the first time in treatment. He is from a middle-class family and lives in a fairly diverse community of working- to middle-class families, but his school is predominantly white. His parents have asked for him to meet with a therapist because of recent issues in school. Edward is a very bright and social child. He is talkative and struggles with staying focused in the classroom. While he maintains generally good grades, he often engages in contentious interactions with teachers because he asks a lot of questions that are perceived as "challenging their authority." Edward's parents, Nicole and Jason, feel concerned about how their son is interacting with authority figures at school. Recently, Edward walked out of class after a teacher told him that if he did not like the way she was teaching, he could leave. For this act, Edward's vice-principal contacted his parents and said that she wanted to meet with them to better understand why he would behave like this, given his good track record at school with no prior disciplinary actions. Following that incident, Edward continued to express frustration with two of his teachers (in his history and finance classes) and was given a verbal warning, placing him at risk of a detention—something that had never happened to him before at school. During conferences, the teachers informed Nicole and Jason that Edward does complete his work, but often responds with information that is outside the scope of what the class is discussing. His history teacher explained that Edward seemed to be "on a mission" to discredit her in the classroom every day. She expressed that she is following the curriculum established by the district, and she understands there may be gaps in it or things left unsaid in the lessons. But students are not allowed to take over the class and start teaching subject matter they have learned elsewhere, she stressed. In the past 2 months since these issues started, Edward has been increasingly angry at home, refusing to do work for both classes, and becoming upset with his parents when they try to force him to do his assignments. They have seen a shift in his usual demeanor and decided to be proactive in requesting therapy for him so he could learn better coping strategies as a young man in a school where he is in the minority and at risk for more scrutiny than other kids. Edward does not believe he needs therapy and notes that he does not understand why his teachers get so annoyed with him.

THERAPIST: Now that I have some general background on what is bringing you into treatment, can you tell me what you suspect may be the issue at school?

EDWARD: I know exactly what it is. The teachers are sometimes teaching us things that I don't think are accurate. They skip a lot of information that I know from watching movies and TikToks and other online sources is not for real. They tell some of the story, but not everything. The only classes where I really have issues are in my history class and sometimes in my one elective class, which is like a financial class I wanted to take.

THERAPIST: Can you give me an example of what happens in one of those classroom situations?

EDWARD: So, I was allowed to sign up for an elective class, and I chose one about finance because I am interested in being a businessperson someday when I am older. In the class one day, the teacher was talking about social economic status and what people from different levels of those statuses make and use money for. So, I asked a question about how it seems like in our county, most of the people at the high level of that range are usually white and if that is true. He kind of stumbled and said no, but that is what is usually the stereotype. Then another kid said that rich African American or Hispanic people are usually musicians or athletes. So, I asked the teacher if that was true and he said he wasn't sure. So, I asked if he could find out because I know a few African American folks in my family that make a lot of money—like maybe not like millions, but they aren't in the middle range like my family, and I think my parents do all right. So, the teacher gets kind of mad and says that is not relevant to what we are talking about. But I was still curious and so the next class, I asked him if he ever got the answers to my questions, and he acted like he couldn't remember. I got frustrated and it turned into a whole thing.

THERAPIST: How has that incident, and the others that you and your parents mentioned, been affecting you lately?

EDWARD: I've just been feeling on edge. Like whenever I go to school and I know those classes are coming up, I feel like I don't know what is going to happen, or if I am going to ask the wrong question. Like, we are going to be talking about what it means to be wealthy and how to invest. I know I am going to want to understand more about why so many African American people who had money at one time had everything taken from them. I learned about the African American Wall Street massacre [1921 Tulsa, Oklahoma, race massacre], and I know that affected a lot of African American people for a long time. And how African American homeowners in cities get their houses bought out from under them, so other people can move in and take over. I learn a lot from my parents and online, and it's like school is teaching something different.

THERAPIST: It sounds like you are saying that you get anxious before these classes because you worry you will ask questions and it will end up with a teacher being mad at you? Is that the feeling, anxiety?

EDWARD: I guess so. I just start thinking about what is going to happen and then what I will say or do, and then what the teacher may say next. It's like I am role playing it out in my mind before

I get there, so I am already amped up and ready for an argument before I even get in that classroom. My teachers say that this always happens and think I am trying to mess up the lesson or make them look bad to the class. But I really just want to learn and figure out where things fit from what I have learned outside of school. I can't help it if other kids laugh or react and make it sound worse than it is.

THERAPIST: That is exactly what feeling anxious can feel like. You are describing it so clearly that I can understand what you are feeling. Let's talk more about this. . . .

Racial Socialization

Like Edward, Nicole, and Jason, Black families have to navigate how to prepare their children for the harsh realities of racism and discrimination, while also helping them to be successful in systems where those issues are embedded. Generations of African American parents in this country have had to walk a line of preparing and teaching without creating a child who is a shrinking violet or resentful. For African American families, socializing children is a rite of passage, rooted in racial trauma going back to enslavement. Enslaved African American parents were in survival mode, developing strategies to navigate an unjust and brutal world. Down through the generations, African American parents have aimed to educate their children about this world and how to survive within it and, in some cases, help to change it. Overall, the racial socialization of African American children is an essential part of child-rearing that is unique, not part of rearing children from other racial groups. This socialization includes education and affirmation in the form of formal and informal messages, preparation for a world where a child will encounter prejudice and discrimination, and practice on how to deal with those issues (Neblitt et al., 2008). Messages shared with African American children that both promote and strengthen racial pride, along with those that help them understand race-based challenges like racism, discrimination, and bias, are a part of the education process. Parents also should aim to affirm their child's sense of self-worth so they are prepared to face these challenges while not internalizing such messages as a reflection of something being wrong with them. And finally, cultural rites of passage like "The Talk" are a part of the preparation and practice that many African American parents engage in to ensure that their child(ren) are equipped with the skills to manage these racial barriers when they occur.

Education

The education for African American children includes messages that promote racial pride, for example, sharing the history of the culture and the many challenges that were overcome, such as enslavement, the Jim Crow era that led to the civil rights movement, and other aspects of history that promote pride in their race. In addition to these messages to promote racial pride, African American parents also focus on teaching their child about racial barriers, such as discrimination and prejudice. This part of a child's education is deemed critical so that they are prepared to face the reality that there are some people who might treat them in unkind and even dangerous ways because of their identity as an African American. Parents may use multiple methods to educate their children to both instill racial pride and to recognize racial barriers through words and actions. Actions may include sharing stories about their own experiences, taking their children to festivals or other events that celebrate African American culture, using music and the arts as a way to promote self-pride and appreciation of their culture. News stories and film may also help drive home messages about racial barriers and help African American youth become aware of situations that happen to Black people because of racism, prejudice, and discrimination.

Affirmation

African American parents may also engage in affirming their child(ren)'s sense of self to promote high self-esteem and self-worth. This is more than just promoting racial pride. Children with a positive sense of self-worth and self-esteem tend to have confidence in their abilities to overcome obstacles and have the resilience to cope when negative life events occur. This aspect of racial socialization is critical because while it does not cancel out the need to be aware of racism and its impact, it helps the child to not internalize this experience and feel as if it is their fault should they be on the receiving end of that discrimination. With a positive sense of self, these children realize that racism is the problem, not them. This echoes the sentiment shared in Part I emphasizing that people are not broken; systems that uphold racist policies and practices are what is broken.

When African American parents in today's world look into the eyes of their children, many of them know that the world is becoming increasingly less predictable and that the world outside of their home may not see their children as innocent, give them room to make a mistake and live to learn from it, or to even be seen as the children they are.

Preparation and Practice

In Nancy Boyd-Franklin's groundbreaking text *Black Families in Therapy: Understanding the African American Experience*, she describes the unique task facing African American parents, who need to equip their children to live in a world that views them with suspicion and provides them with little behavioral wiggle room as they develop (Boyd-Franklin, 2003). This task, a cornerstone of racial socialization, is now commonly referred to as "The Talk." The Talk is a conversation (or maybe more than one) that African American parents have with their children conveying a message about the kinds of interactions that could happen to them when interacting with police officers or other authority figures outside of the home. Through The Talk, parents detail how their children need to conduct themselves in the best way possible to reduce the risk of harm—all the while knowing that even if their children follow those behaviors to the letter, they still may not fare well in such interactions. The Talk has generally, for decades, been just a typical part of the upbringing for many African American children. The appalling social events of recent years mentioned earlier, TV shows like *Black-ish* dedicating a whole episode to the topic, and a widely shown public television advertisement by the Procter & Gamble corporation have made The Talk a part of everyday public discourse.

Preparing to Work with Parents and Children

What is our own cultural identity? In what ways do we understand the experience of African American families, and where do we possibly have hidden spots. Recall the concept of reflective local practice (RLP) that was discussed in Chapter 2. This approach to treatment can help clinicians to better connect with and support African American parents as they help their children—and themselves—navigate a world in which racism and discrimination are so deeply embedded. To use RLP effectively, clinicians must be aware of their own culture and the salient identities they share and do not share with their African American clients. They should also try to acquire knowledge about the unique aspects of their clients' culture and how that informs their values and approaches to child-rearing.

Joining with and Supporting Parents

For African American parents, every time a story like Tamir Rice's is made public, it reinforces the sense of fear, anger, and duty they have to do everything in their power to make sure their children are safe. But what is the burden of carrying that fear, anger, and duty? Parents of African American children should not be on their own when having these conversations with their children. We know that therapy is another avenue to help in the socialization of our clients to the worlds they occupy. We engage in psychoeducation and processing strategies to help people understand their contexts so they can better function in them. And since we know that the impact of racism and discrimination is a stressor that one clinician cannot end, we need to consider how to reduce the burden for parents and increase the resilience and coping strategies of our African American clients to navigate in the world.

To work with African American parents is to help them to process and hold the often-conflicting emotions associated with racial socialization of their children. The dueling experience of having to prepare their children while not scaring them, of having to be specific but also not make sweeping generalizations, and of having to then consider how much or how little to say based on the developmental age and stage of their child—this is not an easy one to navigate. African American parents have been doing this kind of socialization as far back as the days of their ancestors' enslavement. Nevertheless, this child-rearing demand takes an emotional, and consequently physical, toll on parents.

One of the major reasons why African American parents are having to engage in this task of parenting is primarily because no one else will prepare their children for these issues. By educating ourselves as providers, we can now be a part of what trauma therapists Margaret Blaustein and Kristine Kinniburgh (2018) refer to as the "caregiving system." In short, we can become a part of the "village," a reference to the African proverb of it taking a village to raise a child. By sharing in this experience of socializing youth with African American families, clinicians can help to reinforce parents' socializing efforts, but also help them work through the nuances of the anxiety it creates. The intergenerational trauma of racism, and the subsequent practice of socializing African American children, can create elevated fear and resentment that a child may internalize. This could lead to self-hatred and resentment about being African American and what comes with that identity. Instigating this fear and resentment is not what caregivers aim to do in teaching their children, but the risk is there. **Internalized racism** is the result of the development of the belief that being African American is *bad*. It can lead a child to develop behaviors that do not promote pride in who they are, but resistance. That resistance can take the form of constantly feeling compelled to *perform* in ways that do not call attention to themself (based on stereotypical beliefs about African American culture). A child may also try to separate themself from anything (or even anyone) that may call attention to their African American identity, no matter how impossible that is. This is not to be confused with a Black person who happens to have white friends or a white romantic partner. Internalized racism is evident when a person makes an intentional effort to avoid or minimize their identity as an African American because of the shame or fear of how that will be perceived by people of other racial groups.

The Role of Therapists in Supporting African American Parents

Consider the components of racial socialization and where we can map them onto treatment strategies that we already employ. In general, there are four types of messaging that encompass racial socialization:

- Discussions that focus on racial pride
- Preparing the child for discrimination or bias they may encounter
- Promotion of what has often been called a *healthy cultural suspicion* of other racial groups in order to protect oneself—emotionally and physically
- Messages about a youth's individual characteristics as a means to promote a healthy sense of self (Anderson et al., 2021)

Racial socialization is carried out through a set of conversations and assurances that African American parents have with and give to their children, and the skillful behaviors they model for them. There is a certain level of competency in this element of child-rearing that has been shown to reduce anxiety and worry for both the parent *and* their child(ren). Competency in racial socialization skills and confidence can actually be a protective factor for African American children. Racial socialization is a buffer against potential harm, and when it is done with intention, African American parents can feel that having these talks with their children is not a burdensome task that will be met with resentment, but rather messages of empowerment and preparation that can instill realism *and* hope within them. Therapists can help African American parents in the timing and messaging of the racial socialization they do with their children.

So how can clinicians help African American parents, who, for example, might be seeking treatment for their child who is experiencing what Edward did, as described in the vignette that opened this chapter? Most clinicians should approach treatment with certain assumptions:

Assumption 1: Racism and discrimination are not always blatant and obvious to people. It is most damaging in its insidious, vaporous form—embedded in social policy, laws, school curriculum, diagnostic trends, and other systemic factors.

Assumption 2: Most African American families engage in racial socialization of their children, but likely not explicitly calling it that. Parents may not realize that these talks they are having with their children can actually be a protective measure, one that can help their children overcome self-esteem and emotional health issues.

Assumption 3: Everyone has a culture. This is a core element of RLP. When a person recognizes their own salient identities and cultural values, they can be open to hearing about the cultural values and identities of others.

So let's return to the case vignette about Edward and see how the therapist might discuss the matter with his parents, Nicole and Jason.

THERAPIST: Nicole, Edward has shared that he often feels anxious prior to going into his classes, where he has had negative encounters with the teachers. He mentioned that these interactions are due to Edward's questions about possible gaps or misinformation that is being taught in those classrooms. [In this reflective statement, the therapist is creating space for the family to talk more about what the "gaps" or "misinformation" might be. The therapist may have an idea about this, but restating what the client has said in private gives a signal to him that the therapist is open to exploring this issue more fully and willing to hear about it.]

NICOLE: Yes, this is really a problem. And for us, we feel that worry, too. On the one hand, we try to expose him to historical facts that are inclusive of the role of African Americans and speak candidly about racism and discrimination, but we also feel nervous about what happens when he goes into school talking about it when he is one of just a few African American kids in his classes. We don't want him to act like everything they say is the gospel and not ask questions of his teachers, but we also don't want him being perceived as a troublemaker in the classroom and getting into debates with a teacher. It's a catch-22.

JASON: Exactly. Where I think we are struggling is trying to teach him things about our heritage so he can have pride and understand the real world and how we are treated, so he's prepared. But then we don't want him to walk around scared or angry either. It's frustrating to have to hold my breath every day around the time I know he has the history class and the finance class, and have to worry about what might happen or if we are going to get a phone call that something has gone wrong.

THERAPIST: It definitely sounds like you both are having that same kind of anticipatory anxiety about what might happen during these classes. You both are walking that fine line many parents of African American children walk with helping them understand discrimination, racism, and trying to build a sense of pride in all that African Americans have contributed to our nation's history, while also trying to help him navigate school and the fact that there are still major gaps in what we are teaching our children. Is this correct?

In this exchange, the therapist is reflecting what she hears from both parents and is validating the challenge of preparing their child for life both in and out of the classroom. The therapist is also recognizing the anxiety that the challenge is causing. This is an example of how Assumption 1 can help guide the therapist's response, recognizing the ever-present nature of racism and how it affects the family. Labeling this situation as being anxiety-provoking for Jason and Nicole is both normalizing and validating. The process of racial socialization is so deeply embedded in the experience of so many African American families that it may seem novel for a therapist to acknowledge that, while these conversations are necessary and normal in the family, they still produce stress and anxiety that should have space to be processed, if needed.

THERAPIST: The conversations you have been having with Edward are referred to as racial socialization. It's basically the messages that have been passed down through the years from African American parents to their children to help them understand the history of racism and how it affects the way they may be treated. And it also includes instruction on how to handle it. Even though this racial socialization is protective and meant to build Edward's sense of self, it doesn't take away from the natural anxiety you and he feel when he has to head out to school every day. [This feedback offers a formal name to the process of parenting James and Erica are implementing with their child. For many Black families, this is common practice but the term "racial socialization" is not one that is always known to the family. The practice of racial socialization is a custom or culture of parenting passed down through generations. By offering the formal name, as the therapist does here, it is both a moment of psychoeducation, but also normalizes and validates the reward and challenges of this parenting process. This is similar to what can happen when a person is asked to fill out a form related to a particular diagnosis they have received; it feels validating to know that a style of parenting or a way of behaving is so common that is has a name or formal assessment attached to it.]

JASON: So, we didn't know there was a special term for the talks we have been having with him, but yes, it's an odd combination of empowering, frustrating, and scary . . . for him and us, it seems.

THERAPIST: Yes. It will be helpful for us to talk about how you have conveyed messages to Edward and maybe even how you both learned about these things so that you can prepare him. In addition to that, we can talk about helpful strategies for managing the anxiety that comes along with that.

ERICA: I am all for that, but we just don't want my son to have to shrink himself to survive in this school. It's almost like I need him to pick his battles, but still do what he needs to do to be successful in school.

THERAPIST: Absolutely. As a starting point, can you both share more about the things you have talked with Edward about and even where you both recall learning these messages. . . .

In this dialogue, the therapist is expressing curiosity, but also zeroing in on elements of the parents' experience where therapy can be of benefit because it is under their control. When discussing the experience of African American parents, a clinician would be wasting time to try to explain things away, or to make sense of the actions of Edward's teachers. Instead, using specific examples of what Edward and his parents have shared, the clinician can focus on giving the family space in sessions to process their feelings about the areas that feel outside of their control, but also help them develop coping strategies for anxiety and worry. The clinician may consider helping Nicole and Jason navigate how to work with the school and communicate their experience to Edward's teachers, or even join them in advocating on Edward's behalf in the school environment.

Advocacy as a Form of Alliance and Resistance

A powerful role that clinicians can play in helping Black parents who present with their children is to consider more than just building up a sense of resilience within the family. Equally important is being open to stepping into an advocacy role to promote resistance to environments that do not support Black families. Resilience in the therapeutic context usually refers to individual characteristics and skills that help such clients recover from stressful life events. Resistance[1] is more about what a community and its members can do so that individuals do not have to keep going through the process of hurt and recovery (Jones, Anderson, & Stevenson, 2021). Clinicians can play an important role in advocating for a community's efforts to bring about change. When it comes to race-based traumatic stress, disrupting systems is often part of where the healing comes from. Reverend Dr. Martin Luther King Jr. commented on what is most remembered during the fight for civil rights: not the actions of known adversaries, but the silence of those who are supposed to be our friends or allies.

In Edward's case, his current adversity at school is, in part, a function of the teachers' omitting any instruction about the impact of race in the U.S. history of socioeconomic classes and the erasure or minimizing of enslavement and African American contributions to the history of this country. Edward is a child, a student with very little power, yet he is still engaging in what he believes is healthy discourse with his teachers about their stances. The result is that he now is dealing with an anxious mood, distress, and a slow decline in his approach to schoolwork.

---

[1] The use of "resistance" in this context is related to engaging in asserting oneself even when faced with discrimination or prejudiced environments, and not in the therapeutic sense in terms of behaviors that impede therapeutic progress.

Clinicians who aim to help a student in this situation should be willing to consider assuming, as part of their position, an advocacy role on behalf of the student. Such advocacy could involve meeting with Edward's teachers to discuss and educate them about why it is critical that all students in the classroom see the reflection of their culture in the curriculum (beyond just a special month each year). It may also include an offer to provide professional development for school staff about culturally responsive teaching and the psychological impact of a curriculum that reduces cultural groups to a sentence or two for an entire school year.

To that last point, some may feel as if consulting on school curricula will not directly help the family because it is not a direct intervention. However, research about racial socialization suggests that advocacy support for Edward and his parents can help to solidify a therapeutic alliance. Such efforts would also offer additional support to Nicole and Jason, who are likely emotionally exhausted from shouldering the advocacy of their child alone. A therapist's advocacy is not to be mistaken for assuming the family cannot handle the situation. Rather, advocacy is walking the walk of being a culturally responsive provider—a recognition that the root cause of the presenting problem does not lie within the family, but within the system built on and embedded in a history of significant turmoil and discrimination. A mental health clinician from the community willing to come into a school and offer professional development that can help other minority students may be a welcome addition. And even if such outreach is declined by the faculty or school district, the family receiving treatment knows that the clinician is willing to do the work. It would allow Edward's parents to understand that the current state of affairs is not the result of Edward's inability to follow rules or his parents' ability to control his behaviors.

Psychoeducation

Most therapeutic approaches include some element of psychoeducation that helps give labels and meaning to the experiences a family is going through. In the case of Edward, psychoeducation may include discussion about the impact of race-based stress and how it can lead to feelings of anxiety and even emotional exhaustion and frustration. Psychoeducation can be a tool for validating and normalizing the experiences of Black children and families. It would also be relevant for a clinician to share information about how stress and trauma, when experienced over long stretches, can even result in symptoms similar to those of PTSD (e.g., avoidance of triggers, poor concentration, sleep disturbance).

Relevant and Accessible Coping Skills

Anderson, McKenny, and Stevenson (2019) describe a model that helps to reduce race-based traumatic stress through specific and targeted racial socialization interventions between parents and their children. This model, called Engaging, Managing, and Bonding through race (EMBrace), includes a discussion of the importance of offering reflective exercises that can help clients cope with the stress of various types of encounters, like those that Edward and his family are dealing with. Activities such as journaling, relaxation strategies, engaging in artistic hobbies that allow for self-expression are just some examples of helping individuals lean into and process their emotions. This behavior is preferable to the avoidant strategies of withdrawing and isolating, what Edward began to do as he became more frustrated with his schoolteachers and curriculum issues. It would also be helpful to encourage the family members to engage in coping strategies at the same time in order for them to bond and manage their stress linked to racial discrimination together. This can be daily mantras or affirmations before leaving home, or making space each evening to talk about how their day went and what they might need to do to recover from whatever stressors had occurred. Affirmations and mantras are strategies for building a sense of self that can then become the internal dialogue to help override feelings of dismissal and minimizing, just like those affecting Edward at school.

Another coping strategy that clinicians can explore with Black parents and families is to tap into the family's spiritual faith. As outlined in the works of Boyd-Franklin (2013), Turner et al. (2019), Parker et al. (2023), and many other sources, spirituality plays a complex role in the lives of African Americans, and in their understanding of mental illness and seeking of mental health treatment. Although there are vast differences among African Americans in terms of their religious practices and denominations of faith, spirituality, beliefs rooted in faith, and reliance on a higher power can play a role in their perceptions of how they should raise and seek help for their children. A clinician may consider introducing this topic by asking about what, if any, role the family's spirituality plays in their life and then expand the conversation to include topics related to how it ties to their expectations of themselves, their children, and how it affects them. In doing so, the therapist may be able to help the family identify ways that their spirituality can become a strength to rely on, to help persevere through the challenges that have led them to treatment.

>   THERAPIST: We have talked a bit about your child(ren)'s areas of strengths and needs. I am curious about other aspects of your family's life. What are some of your family values, beliefs, etc.? What are some important foundational beliefs you have, if any?
>
>   PARENT: Well, my wife and I were both raised in the church, but we do not go as religiously any more. A lot has changed, so while we still try to share with the kids those foundational principles of our faith, we don't go to a formal church as often as I did when I was growing up.
>
>   THERAPIST: What are some of those foundational principles that you teach to your children? [This open question gives the client room to expand his thinking and ponder what exact principles have resonated enough with him and his wife that they are choosing to share them with their children.]
>
>   PARENT: Well, like telling the truth, standing up for others who can't stand up for themselves, doing the right thing, even when it is hard or unpopular, things like that. We just try to teach them that they should pray, show gratitude, and just be good people. They are in a world that doesn't always treat people who look like us in a positive way. I want them to be strong internally so that they don't rely on the opinions or prejudices of others to tear down their self-esteem.

A conversation like this can help a clinician gain insight into how faith and spiritual practice can be used to fortify the self-esteem of, and give affirmation to, a Black person or family. While discussions of faith can be helpful with clients regardless of race, the literature cited above speaks to the elevated role that spirituality has in the willingness or reticence of Black people to pursue mental health services. And for Black parents, discussions of spirituality add to the overall dialogue about racial socialization. Prayer and seeking circles of support in church are ways in which Black parents may cope with their concerns and fears about how their children are being affected by racism and discrimination. Clinicians who are providing culturally responsive care to African Americans would be remiss to exclude any inquiry about the role that spirituality may play in their parenting and relationships.

Building Racial Competency Skills

For African American parents, the stress and worry of raising children often revolve around their need to feel confident that they are adequately preparing their sons and daughters for a world that may treat them with much bias and prejudice. Clinicians working with Black families should be knowledgeable and willing to discuss how the family approaches racial socialization. For clinicians who may not have shared lived experience with the family, gaining this knowledge is even more important. Regardless of the clinician's racial/ethnic identity, the use of measures can facilitate conversations about parenting and socialization. For example, the Racial Socialization Competency Scale (RaSCS; Anderson, Jones, & Stevenson, 2020) can be a useful tool for practitioners working with Black families to get a sense of the families' confidence, skills, and stress related to providing racial socialization messages to their children and modeling adaptive coping behavior for them. The items on this measure may help facilitate discussion with parents in therapy sessions. Also, for many clients, no matter their race, when a clinician offers a measure related to their presenting concerns, that in and of itself can feel validating because the existence of a formal model indicates that many other people face these same concerns. The RaSCS has items that the respondent endorses, such as "I share my emotions about my experiences of racial encounters," "I teach my child to share their feelings about the history of racism and slavery." In the case of Edward's parents, this kind of measure can help the clinician identify areas where they feel more or less confident or stressed, and help them consider different strategies to support Edward while maintaining his sense of hope and optimism, in spite of how his teachers respond to his questions at school.

While African American families are not a monolith and differing salient factors impact their emotional health, clinicians only benefit the therapeutic experience by increasing their own awareness of racial socialization in Black families. This awareness can improve their ability to connect with the underlying forces impacting the families they treat, especially when they are functioning in environments that often uphold policies and procedures deeply embedded in racism and discrimination. So many African American families have been taught—implicitly and explicitly—that the biases and prejudices that they may encounter are a normal part of their lives. They have been taught to be aware of and manage experiences of prejudice to the best of their ability. But we know now that managing these experiences "effectively" can come at a cost. The emotional and physical impact of race-based traumatic stress is well documented and covered in other chapters in this book, but it is important for clinicians to increase their comfort with inviting discussion about this subject into the therapeutic space. It can be a part of formulating an alliance with the client and affirm that the clinician is a person who is comfortable discussing uncomfortable topics like racism and discrimination.

CHAPTER TAKEAWAYS

- Racial socialization is a part of child-rearing for many African American families. While not always explicitly labeled as such, it is important to note that this form of socialization has been passed down through generations as a form of teaching Black children survival skills for recognizing and managing racism and discrimination in their everyday world. Clinicians should educate themselves on this practice and talk to African American families about how they share those messages and the impact they believe it may have on their family functioning.

- The clinician can serve as an advocate for families so that they do not have to bear the burden of addressing biased systems on their own. In doing so, the clinician takes a step further than simply helping individuals tap into their own resilience; rather, they become an active participant in resistance—disrupting systems that are upholding practices steeped in racism and white supremacy.

- Clinicians should recognize their cultural similarities and differences with clients and be open to discussing where they may have less knowledge. This might help put families at ease because they know the clinician is open to hearing from them and is not placing themself in the position of sole expert in the room.

PART III
HEALING FROM RACIAL TRAUMA

CHAPTER 8

Healer, Heal Me
Healing Clients from Racial Trauma

> Freeing yourself was one thing, claiming ownership
> of that freed self was another.
> —TONI MORRISON (1987, p. 426)[1]

Toya[2] is a 24-year-old African American cisgender woman who informs her white cisgendered psychologist that she is experiencing some anxiety because she just found out she is pregnant. Toya has three children (4- and 6-year-old boys and a 2-year-old girl). She was in the process of separating from the children's father who had already moved out, but kept seducing her when he visited them. Toya has been in therapy with this psychologist for a few weeks.

TOYA: I feel really stressed, but also happy and blessed. I know things will work out. My spiritual being tells me that I will be OK. Although . . . I just did not expect this pregnancy now.

---

[1] Excerpt from *Beloved* by Toni Morrison. Copyright © 1987 by Toni Morrison. Used by permission of Alfred A. Knopf, an imprint of the Knopf Doubleday Publishing Group, a division of Penguin Random House LLC. All rights reserved.

[2] This example was developed by Lucy Takagi, PsyD, LLC, for the 2019 NJPA Fall Conference. The case was inspired by reports from actual patients, described in the 2018 dissertation of Mercedes Jean Okosi, PsyD: "The Impact of Racial Microaggressions in the Therapeutic Relationships with People of Color" at the Graduate School of Applied and Professional Psychology (GSAPP).

PSYCHOLOGIST: Yes, it seems quite a surprise. You already have three children, correct?

TOYA: Yes, two boys and one girl. They keep my hands full (*smiling*).

PSYCHOLOGIST: I see. And their father is already out of the home, correct?

TOYA: He is out of the home, but he visits us.

PSYCHOLOGIST: Since you seemed to be getting intimate with him during his visits, did you take precautions to prevent the pregnancy?

TOYA: Yes. I did. I cannot take pills, but we used condoms every time. I know it is not 100% safe, but I thought I was protecting myself.

PSYCHOLOGIST: I see. Do you think that maybe a part of you could have wanted to get pregnant?

TOYA: Not that I am aware of.

PSYCHOLOGIST: Well, sometimes we do things without being necessarily aware of the reasons why. I wonder if there was a part of you that did not see a problem with having many children. . . .

TOYA: (*pause*) I love my children. They were born out of my love for their father. That love is not the way it was, but we still love each other. . . . We just can't live with each other.

PSYCHOLOGIST: What about the children? Have you thought of them?

TOYA: What do you mean?

PSYCHOLOGIST: I am just wondering if you considered what it is like for the children, to have a mama who is rarely there because she has to work all the time to keep food on the table.

TOYA: But I am there.

PSYCHOLOGIST: I see.

TOYA: (*getting annoyed*) I am not sure what you are getting at. I am there for my children. And I will be there for this one, too. I love them. I am a good mother, just like my mother was a good mother to me and my grandmother was a great mother to her. I know I am a good mother. I am just anxious because this pregnancy was unexpected, but I will manage it. It will be OK. I will talk to my pastor and get some help. It will be OK.

PSYCHOLOGIST: It seems like you got angry at me when all I attempted to do Toya was to explore how your children would feel with a new sibling. I am wondering if that anger is misdirected.

TOYA: I am not angry, but I am getting annoyed. It seems you are blaming me for this pregnancy. All I said was that I was stressed and, yes, I am stressed because I just found out I will have a fourth child, without having planned for it. I guess I have some reason to feel stressed.

PSYCHOLOGIST: Yes.

TOYA: Anyway. The children's father said he will help and support me financially. He has been supportive since he moved out. I also can continue to work until I am close to my due date, and my family can help me. I guess I will be OK.

PSYCHOLOGIST: It seems like you are trying to convince yourself that you will.

TOYA: Yeah, I guess . . .

PSYCHOLOGIST: Have you considered other alternatives?

TOYA: Like what?

PSYCHOLOGIST: I do not want you to misunderstand me. I am not trying to tell you to do anything. As your psychologist, I need to help you explore all possibilities. You tell me you are stressed and that you did not expect this pregnancy. You are separated from the children's father. Have you considered terminating this pregnancy?

TOYA: I would never do that. Actually, I am shocked you raised that as a possibility. I know you are supposed to question me, but I get the sense that you disapprove of this pregnancy and that instead of helping me with my anxiety, you are making it worse.

PSYCHOLOGIST: (*quiet*)

TOYA: (*in a firm and controlled tone*) I am wondering if we could talk about how you as a middle-class white psychologist can judge my pregnancy. I came here for soul care and am getting blamed for being pregnant.

PSYCHOLOGIST: Toya, I believe you might have misunderstood me. I did not blame you. I attempted to explore your reasons for being anxious about this pregnancy, which is my job. Somehow, it seems that you are getting angry or even furious at me. I am interested in understanding why, but unless you take a deep breath and calm yourself, this conversation will not be productive.

TOYA: OK, I was not angry with you when we started this conversation, but now I am. You seem to be doing what other white people do, pegging me as an angry Black woman, instead of listening to what I am experiencing. You are pegging me as a Black woman who did nothing to prevent her pregnancy and who should not have a fourth child. I honestly believe that is my prerogative and not yours. And when I confront that, you peg me as an angry Black woman.

PSYCHOLOGIST: Toya, this has nothing to do with race or class. This has to do with how difficult it is for you to recognize that your life seems to be getting out of control. Three little children, a separation, another pregnancy—these are the topics we are discussing. Race did not enter into the equation.

TOYA: But race is ALWAYS in the equation for me!

PSYCHOLOGIST: Help me understand.

TOYA: NO! You find a way to understand it yourself. I should not have come to talk to a white woman about being stressed. I am strong. I should have known better. Have a good day!

As we have made clear earlier in the book, racial trauma is the stressful impact or emotional pain of one's experience with racism, discrimination, and racial violence. The reactions to this trauma reflect injury to a person, not a mental illness. These injuries are invisible wounds held deeply by individuals, groups, and communities. When racial trauma injuries go unaddressed, there can be lasting mental, emotional, and physical health issues. One does not just get over a trauma. The impact of the trauma needs to be acknowledged, believed, and affirmed to open the door to healing.

To become truly competent at providing therapy in the face of racial trauma, it is important to recognize the distinction between Eurocentric and Black/African psychology. Black/African psychology is a subfield of psychology that challenges Eurocentric psychology. The discipline of psychology is defined as the study of behavior and the mind. Eurocentric psychologists' aim is for the discipline of psychology to be viewed as a science, specifically as a STEM (science, technology, engineering, mathematics) subject. For psychology to be a science, there is an abundance of emphasis on the use of the scientific method as a means to collect, analyze, and interpret empirical data. Conversely, Black/African psychologists have long challenged this paradigm and approach to psychology. African psychology posits that the nature of knowledge construction is not limited to the tangible, or that which is observable (Cokley & Garba, 2018).

Black psychology is viewed as understanding the lifestyles of Black people based on their authentic experiences in this country (White, 1970). In contrast, African-centered psychology is concerned with defining African psychological experiences from an African perspective. These psychological experiences reflect an African orientation to the meaning of life, the world, and relationships with others and oneself (Grills & Ajie, 2002). Black/African psychology values self-knowledge and intuition as equally important sources of knowledge. It defines the nature of reality and understands human behavior in distinctly different ways from those of traditional Eurocentric psychology (Grills & Ajie, 2002). In the article "Speaking Truth to Power: How Black/African Psychology Changed the Discipline of Psychology," Cokley and Garba (2018) explained how historically Black psychologists were constantly exposed to messages of Black deficiency, pathology, and inferiority. Joseph White's pivotal "Toward a Black Psychology" was the first article to articulate an authentic, non-deficit-based psychology for Black people (White, 1970). In this article, White argued that psychology frequently and wrongly described Black individuals as lacking or deviant because it relied on Eurocentric norms to understand behavior.

Understanding Black/African psychology, how it vastly differs from Eurocentric psychology, is key to understanding how to heal Black people from racially traumatic events. If we view Black individuals as the holder of the problem, which is how Eurocentric psychology has traditionally described psychopathology, then we think of racial trauma as something that can be "fixed" in the individual rather than "healed."

Why use foundations and aspects of Black culture when addressing racial harms and wounds? Because culture cures, culture protects, culture promotes resiliency, and culture fosters self-awareness. As noted earlier, there is a difference between coping with racially charged events and healing from them. Coping skills are the thoughts and behaviors we use to manage stressful situations. Healing is the process of becoming sound or healthy again.

Affirming a client's personal strengths and replacing negative beliefs can help them heal from racialized trauma. Healing also means involving the community and helping the client to realize that they are not the only ones coping. Increasing the client's sense of belonging can counter their sense that they are alone in feelings and experiences triggered by racialized trauma.

Individual Healing

Christopher is a 16-year-old Black male in therapy with the encouragement of his mother and art teacher. About a year ago, Christopher moved to a predominately white neighborhood with his family and is having a difficult time adjusting. He is a talented artist and spends his free time working with his art teacher doing projects around the school, and even around the town he lives in. His mother noticed Christopher becoming more and more angry, and having outbursts over little things. For example, he came home 30 minutes late one evening, and when his mother attempted to address this with him, he exploded and yelled (not at her but in general) that people always think he is doing something wrong. His art teacher also noticed that over the past year he has become short-tempered. His anger is never directed at anyone, but he explodes by yelling when trying to defend his actions. He agreed to see a therapist to address this issue because he also did not want to be so angry all of the time. By his third session, he began highlighting the possible root cause of his anger. He said,

> "Dr. C, it's crazy out here being Black in a white neighborhood. Everybody looks at me all the time everywhere I go, like I'm an alien and I am about to do something wrong. I mean, I go into a store with my friends downtown and no matter what, everyone

is looking at me like I'm going to rob the store. The lady behind the desk always has her eyes on me. I see the looks. I know the looks because they happen all the time. I hate living in a white neighborhood because no one looks like me. I can go a whole day without seeing another person like me. It's like I always have to prove I'm not going to rob them. I'm not going to trash the place. I'm not going to hurt them. I'm just buying something to drink like everybody else. I just want to scream and tell them all to just leave me the hell alone, but I'm not an idiot. I know I can't say anything to them folks [*white people*] because the minute I try to explain myself, that lady is going to feel 'threatened' and the next thing you know, she starts screaming and yelling, then the police come, and the next thing you know, I'm on the ground with my hands behind my back or worse shot and killed by the police all because I was trying to tell her to stop staring at me because I'm not doing anything wrong."

In his 2013 article "Healing the Hidden Wounds of Racial Trauma," Kenneth Hardy lays out eight key steps for healing when working with people of color: (1) affirmation and acknowledgment, (2) create space for race, (3) racial storytelling, (4) validation, (5) the process of naming, (6) externalized devaluation, (7) counteract devaluation, and (8) rechanneling rage. These steps are a useful jumping off point when conducting therapy with individuals who are dealing with the repercussions of racialized events in their lives—because they address the many aspects of the individual and validates their experiences.

Being a Black youth, Christopher is exposed to racially injurious and sometimes traumatizing conditions every day. Using Dr. Hardy's eight key steps to addressing racial trauma, we will walk through the case of Christopher.

Affirmation and acknowledgment involves the counselor helping the client develop a sense of understanding and acceptance of racial issues. It is important for the counselor to convey the premise that race is a critical organizing principle in society. The counselor can say something like, "Everywhere you go, you will always be Black; there is no ignoring that and what that means to you in this society. When you go to school, you are Black. When you walk in a store, you are Black. Being Black will always factor in how you interact in society and how society interacts with you, for good or bad." While Christopher understands that, it has been difficult for him. He is a Black male in a white neighborhood with people around him who do not recognize or acknowledge how hard this is. The therapist's role is to affirm Christopher's racial experiences and acknowledge that they are having an impact on him. This is possible because a foundation was established early in therapy that allowed the therapist and Christopher to openly talk about race and racial issues. If for some reason such a foundation is not set in the beginning of the counselor's work with a client, the counselor can still introduce the topic of race as their work evolves.

As an example, the counselor might say, "We don't usually talk about race in therapy, but I've been wondering how being Black in a predominately white town has been impacting you lately?" Christopher may respond, "No one has ever asked me that before. It's so hard being the only Black person in so many spaces. I wish I had a few more friends that were Black so we could all stick together and someone else would get what I am going through." If the counselor does not identify as Black, they could offer, "Although I am not Black and can't possibly know what you might be going through, I want you to know that I am open to hearing anything you need to say right now about how being Black in a white neighborhood is impacting you." Christopher's response might be "Thank you, I wasn't sure if I could talk about race in here because I don't want to offend you, but being Black in an all-white neighborhood is so hard on me." Through this affirmation and acknowledgment, the counselor can allow conversations about race to emerge in a safe and nonthreatening way.

Creating a space for race allows for an open dialogue with clients. Hardy notes that we must take a proactive role to identify race as a significant variable and talk openly about experiences related to race. When working with Christopher, the therapist encouraged him to talk openly and candidly about his experiences of being Black. This led to his recounting of his daily life.

>   THERAPIST: Tell me what it's like when you go out with your friends.
>
>   CHRISTOPHER: Well, you know, we hang out and listen to music. Sometimes we may go to the mall and just walk around.

THERAPIST: Does your Blackness ever come up with your friends? Remember, it is OK to talk about race and how you're feeling being the only Black person in your group of friends.

CHRISTOPHER: Only sometimes. Like when we are listening to music sometimes, they think I will know all the words to the rap songs. . . . I actually do (*he laughs*) but no one asks Joey, or Mike, or even JJ who knows all the words like I do. I think they ask me because I am Black. Sometimes it's no big deal, but other times it's like I just stand out.

THERAPIST: How does that impact you . . . standing out among your friends?

CHRISTOPHER: It makes me stay in my head all the time. It's like I can't even just relax and just chill with them. I'm in my head missing my friends from my old neighborhood. Sometimes I think they just want to be my friend because it's cool to be the Black guy's friend.

THERAPIST: So, you are self-conscious around them.

CHRISTOPHER: Yeah, that's it. I don't want to be self-conscious, I just want to chill and relax like everyone else.

THERAPIST: How does it feel to talk about this with me?

CHRISTOPHER: It feels good that somebody gets it. My mom always tries to tell me that I'll fit in soon, just give it time. But I don't want to fit in. I want to be me and not have to worry that being me is going to make me stand out all the time!

In addition to open dialogue—when we take creating a space for race a step further—the therapist should think about the physical environment where clients come for therapy. When developing a space for Black clients to receive treatment, know that the physical environment sets the tone as clients enter the building. Being mindful of comfortable furnishings, artwork, plants, magazines/books, and personal memorabilia is important. Moreover, a therapist can consider all these aspects of their office from a cultural standpoint.

Racial storytelling is a technique whereby the counselor invites the client to share their personal stories of racial experiences. The counselor's role here is to guide clients into thinking critically about their experiences around being Black. These experiences can fall on a spectrum from positive to negative. With Christopher, he was focused on the negative aspects of being Black. He often mentioned that being Black meant sticking out in a crowd, and not in a good way. He believed that the very essence of being Black would always subject him to suspicion from others. It is true that in one aspect of his life he feels scrutinized because of his skin color. Yet, there are other stories he had yet to tell that celebrated his Blackness in powerful ways.

During one session, the therapist took some time to guide him through encounters where he was proud to be Black. This technique allowed him to see himself in ways he never allowed. His first story involved feeling proud when another Black person in his life persevered. He recounted attending his cousin's high school graduation when he was 11 and seeing his cousin Michael on the stage because he had been named the class valedictorian. He described seeing his cousin sitting onstage in a sea of white faces (principal, superintendent, teachers, salutatorian) and thought to himself how proud he was of Michael. When the therapist pressed Christopher further and asked him what about that moment made him proud to be Black, he sat back and responded, "Michael was the only Black person on that stage, and he was getting the highest honor. Something in me just smiled and being Black in that moment felt like everything." This was a great opportunity to connect that story to his own reality of being one of a few Black students in his current school and highlighting what it would feel like to be proud of being Black in white spaces. This storytelling technique gave Christopher a voice to create his own narrative around being Black.

Validation offers confirmation of the client's worldview and self-worth. In other words, it is an opportunity to counter what Hardy calls "internalized devaluation," when a Black individual internalizes societal beliefs that whiteness is superior to Blackness, which is a direct byproduct of racism. When Christopher shared his heartbreaking experiences in the store (where he was believed to be up to no good and likely a threat), it was crucial that his therapist validate his experiences. The therapist purposely pointed out and validated who Christopher actually was in this situation. He was not a criminal. He was not a thug. He was not someone there to cause others harm. The therapist told Christopher that he was a 16-year-old young Black man who managed to control his emotions and show restraint in the midst of harmful microaggressions. Validation is an opportunity for the therapist to go one step further from acknowledging race—an organizing principal in society—and provide confirmation of a client's own racial identity, worldview, and self-worth.

Naming racial experiences is the next step. In the year 2020, the world faced an unknown virus that was taking the lives of millions. It was named COVID-19, and by naming the virus, we knew what we had to fight. Naming the virus, examining it, and figuring out how it operated and impacted people allowed us to finally combat it. If the virus had no name and there was no common language to discuss where it came from, how it operated, and its impact, then there would have been no way to manage the virus. Racism, **racial oppression**, microaggressions, macroassaults, and racial trauma in recent years have all been clearly defined and their impact is palpable (see the end-of-book Glossary). If these concepts were to remain nameless, difficult to describe, measure, or classify, they would go unexamined and unaddressed. Naming a problem like racial trauma, especially when some folks do not even believe it exists, is a powerful action. Therefore, the major objective for the therapist at this step is to ascribe words to racially based experiences and to give these words meanings. Imagine how difficult it is for a client to try to describe their experiences and not have the words to do so. It feels isolating and lonely because they may think that this is something only happening to them. It is difficult for a client to grasp they have been significantly impacted by something that does not even have a name. Therefore, name these experiences so they can be examined and addressed.

Christopher was an artist. When he did not have words, he had his sketches and paintings. Words to describe his experiences were often elusive for him. He knew he was angry, but he had difficulty expressing (naming) what was behind the anger. As he recounted stories from his daily life, it was important for Christopher to have a language that described his experiences. He learned what a microaggression was for the first time in therapy. He had heard the term "profiling" used before but was taken aback when he and the therapist explored the difference between profiling and "racial profiling," and how that felt when it happened to him. Christopher was slowly finding his voice to describe his experiences, which led him to develop the ability to describe the impact of these experiences.

> THERAPIST: (*in reference to his recounting of browsing at the store and being stared at*) What you described to me was racial profiling. We can't read her mind and know why the woman was staring at you, but when we put all the pieces together, you felt she was staring because you were the only Black person in the store.
>
> CHRISTOPHER: So, what happened to me was racial profiling?
>
> THERAPIST: Yes, you were being singled out as she assumed you were doing something wrong based on your appearance. Your outward appearance is that of a Black teenage male. You were with your friends who are white teenage males, and they were not being profiled. Race-based profiling relies on stereotypes of racial or ethnic groups.
>
> CHRISTOPHER: Wow, what you are saying makes sense. I never have the words to explain what is happening to me. So, I can't explain it to my mom or Ms. Brown (*his art teacher*). Everyone thinks I'm angry for no reason, but I have reasons. I just didn't know how to explain it.

Externalizing devaluation is a way for the client to recognize that racialized events do not define them or their self-worth. The goal is to increase their respect for themself despite negative outside racial messaging.

The therapist needed to assist Christopher with recognizing that racially traumatic events do not define him. He gets the opportunity to define who he is and what kind of person he wants to be. Through therapy, Christopher was learning to recognize that the disrespect he was encountering in various spaces was connected to race and racial oppression. His yelling outbursts, his anger, stemmed from a yearning for respect in spaces where he felt as if he was not getting any. This anger was bleeding over into his relationships with loved ones who truly valued and respected him. Here, the goal for Christopher was for him to recognize that racial assaults do not lessen his self-worth.

CHRISTOPHER: I don't know why I'm angry all the time and always yelling at my mom when she tells me to do things. I don't mean to yell, but I'm so frustrated with everyone telling me what to do and how to act.

THERAPIST: Who is everyone? Who is telling you how to act?

CHRISTOPHER: Everyone is—my mom, my teachers, shoot . . . even myself.

THERAPIST: What do you mean by "even myself"?

CHRISTOPHER: I have to be a different me in some spaces. I have to do things to fit in and not stand out. Like when I am in my honors English class, I have to speak differently because the teacher is always correcting my words. She calls it slang, and I call it the way I talk. So, I make an extra effort to speak the way the other guys are speaking, so I don't stand out.

THERAPIST: What you are describing is code switching.

CHRISTOPHER: What's that?

THERAPIST: **Code switching** is the way a Black person, or someone from an underrepresented group, consciously or unconsciously adjusts their language, behavior, and appearance to fit into the white culture.

CHRISTOPHER: Yes, I do that all the time! I can't be who I am. I feel worthless as myself in school and in this damn town.

THERAPIST: These events do not define you. You get to define who you are. Code switching can be seen as a way to survive a world created and maintained by the dominant culture . . . I mean the white culture. You are worth more than these experiences. Remember that!

Counteracting devaluation provides clients with resources that help to rebuild their emotional, psychological, and behavioral well-being in the wake of racial assaults. Dr. Martin Luther King Jr. said, "Somebody told a lie one day . . . they made everything Black ugly and evil." These constant messages of Black inferiority are difficult to ward off if our clients do not have the tangible resources to do so. It was vital to Christopher's healing to face these messages that were assaulting and debilitating him. To do this, Christopher worked hard on changing the narrative that was playing in his head, telling him he was not good enough.

> CHRISTOPHER: Dr. C, it's like I'm not good enough anywhere I go. Even my teachers seem surprised that I answer questions right.
>
> THERAPIST: Where do you think that voice, "I'm not good enough," comes from?
>
> CHRISTOPHER: I guess from me 'cause I'm just not good enough . . . like I said, anywhere I go.
>
> THERAPIST: From what you're telling me, you may be getting the message you are not good enough from the people and places around you. You are getting constant messages that you are not good enough. When you go to the store, the store clerk thinks you are not good enough to shop in her store. When you're in school, you mentioned the teachers are surprised you are very intelligent. You are internalizing these messages, and they are not true. You are good enough, more than good enough. When that thought comes into your head, work hard to catch it and remind yourself that you are what you are meant to be and that is a valuable person.

These constant messages from people in Christopher's environment were undermining his sense of self. Through this therapy that aimed to counter devaluation, Christopher learned to look at aspects of his life that challenged such narratives, and he worked hard to create a new narrative.

Rechanneling rage is the final step in Hardy's approach to healing the hidden wounds of racial trauma. Rage comes in many forms, but the result can be self-destructive. The rage comes from not having a voice in one's experiences and feelings of powerlessness in one's own life. The writer James Baldwin once said, "To be a negro in this country and to be relatively conscious is to be in a rage almost all of the time" (Baldwin et al., 1961, p. 205). Rage should be normalized as a reasonable or predictable reaction to abnormal events. However, staying in a rage all the time is not healthy. There are long-term mental and physical effects of anger: anxiety, high blood pressure, and headaches, to name just a few.

Christopher had a right to be angry and even in a rage over his experiences. His issue was that he felt this anger surfaced during the most inopportune moments. The goal of Christopher's treatment was not to get rid of his anger. The goal was to understand its origins and discuss the usefulness of this anger. Using the step of rechanneling rage, Christopher was learning to gain control over his emotions and not let his anger consume him. Additionally, he and his therapist worked on redirecting his anger away from those closest to him who are not causing him harm.

Healing as a Community

On June 17, 2015, a white man named Dylan Roof walked into a historic African American church and asked for the pastor. After finding the pastor, he sat down next to him and participated in the church's bible study. At its end, the bible study participants stood, bowed their heads, and began to pray. It was at this time that Dylan Roof pulled a gun from his fanny pack and shot and killed nine members of the Mother Emanuel AME Church including the pastor.

The following Sunday, 750 miles away, a small Black Baptist church was filled with members whose sentiments were "We are not even safe in our place of worship." The members of this small congregation did not know the members or victims from Mother Emanuel, yet the fear for their own safety was palpable. One congregant at this Baptist church told me (J. R. J.-D.), "Every time that back door opened in the sanctuary, I shuttered and prayed that I recognized the person coming through the door." The members of this church were experiencing vicarious racial trauma and were at a loss to explain what that term even meant and how to address it.

The Association of Black Psychologists (ABPsi) collaborated with the Community Healing Network to create Emotional Emancipation Circles (EECs). EECs were created so communities might heal from within. Instead of an outside counselor coming in, facilitating groups, and conducting individual therapy, the EECs were created to empower the people to take control of their own healing. The role of the counselor is to empower members of a community with the tools that are already at their fingertips. These tools can seem elusive at first, but the counselor can ignite a fire in a community that needs no assistance with shining brightly. It is a powerful thing when a community comes together and heals from within.

The small Black church in the case study here was given the tools to facilitate their own EECs. The purpose was to address their pain and trauma from the racial incidents the church's members had experienced as individuals, those experienced by the church itself, and the most recent racial trauma experienced vicariously and collectively in the wake of the shooting at Mother Emanuel. EECs became a space where these church members could come together and share their stories, deepen their understanding of the impact of racial events on their emotions and relationships, and learn and practice emotional wellness skills. The goal was to have the small Black church recognize their interdependence by practicing cooperation, self-discipline, sacrifice, and unconditional love. Through these practices, the church would foster stronger families, community, and unbreakable people.

An additional culturally grounded crisis response program created by the ABPsi to interrupt the stress and racial trauma responses of Black individuals is the Sawubona Healing Circles. These circles are virtual or in-person safe spaces for individuals of African ancestry that draw on culturally grounded healing strategies in coping with anti-Black racial trauma/stress and community violence. The circles are not intended to be therapy or a replacement for therapy if it is needed. The Sawubona Healing Circles are supportive and culturally affirming spaces to promote wellness and overall social–emotional adjustment. The outcomes include participants learning principles of cultural wisdom and protective factors to assist in coping with racial stress.

The term *Sawubona* is a Zulu phrase that means "I see you" or "We see you." This Zulu greeting is more than words of politeness. Sawubona stresses the importance of recognizing the worth and dignity of each person. Using an African-centered worldview, these circles recognize and validate racial traumas and stressors that people of African descent experience; these circles equip them with African-centered healing (Auguste et al., 2024). The goal of Sawubona Healing Circles assists

Black communities in stepping out of ordinary stressful times and into a safe and accepting environment with other Black-identified individuals where they can explore their healing. These circles are also ideal for incidences that lead to the need for community healing.

As a counselor, launching a communitywide intervention is no small feat. The first step is to find a clearly defined community. In the case of the small Black church, what made them a community was membership in the church, and the love and support of each other. Once the community has been defined, find stakeholders within the community that can engage and inspire participants. With open minds, everyone works together to discover the best ways to remove obstacles to healing, alleviate suffering, and deepen their capacity to heal. Unless you are a part of the community, your goal is to have the healing process led by someone within the community. Remember, there is strength in healing coming from within the community and not from an outside source.

CHAPTER TAKEAWAYS

- There is a risk of retraumatizing the client by ignoring or not recognizing their perception of racial trauma or racially charged events that have impacted them. At times, there is a desire to debate the client's perception of trauma and racism. Be sure to allow time and space for your client to express their anger at racism. Also, do not assume that all Black people will perceive racism in a given situation. Their presenting issues when entering therapy may seem far away from any racialized events. A therapist must remember the context in which all the client's problems are embedded: a society that is filled with racism and devalues Black lives.

- The therapist should remind themselves about the difference between coping with racially adverse events and healing from them. Black individuals are resilient, and within their stories are a host of strengths from which they can draw when they encounter racialized events. The story they are telling the counselor now is most likely not the first time they encountered a racialized event that had an impact on them. Therefore, questions such as "How have you overcome traumatic experiences in the past?" or "How have you dealt with racist events in your life?" are great starting points to highlight resilience and strengths. Keep at the forefront of your mind the historic resilience of Black people.

- Empathy and understanding are keys to acknowledging racial hurt and putting the client on the path of healing. Remember to be emotionally present with clients, sit with them in what they are going through, and try to understand the client's perspective. Allow clients to share their stories and refrain from debating whether racism was involved.

CHAPTER 9

Healer, Heal Thyself
Vicarious Racial Trauma and Self-Care

> As soon as healing takes place, go out
> and heal somebody else.
> —MAYA ANGELOU (1997)

Krystal Morris was a Black-identified newly licensed psychologist working at a community counseling center at the height of the COVID-19 pandemic in 2020. Then the murder of George Floyd ricocheted throughout the country and the world. Dr. Morris watched the video of George Floyd being murdered and was dealing with her own feelings and reactions in response to that. At this time, more Black-identified clients sought therapy and called the counseling center. Dr. Morris's supervisor decided it would be beneficial for these new Black-identified clients to be connected to a Black therapist. Therefore, without Dr. Morris's input, her caseload grew from racially mixed to primarily individuals who identified as Black. After 6 weeks of listening to her clients' stories and the impact the racial events had on them, Dr. Morris felt herself becoming overwhelmed and even helpless at times. She had barely had a chance to process everything herself before having to process the feelings of her clients with them. She often thought to herself, "But . . . I'm in pain too." Dr. Morris called in sick to work more often, had physical reactions such as increased headaches, and was emotionally exhausted every day. She began to lose joy in helping others and considered resigning from the counseling center.

Escaping the imagery of Black individuals being hurt, harmed, or killed because of their race can be nearly impossible. We live in a world of constant news cycles and social media that provide us with updates on almost any event in moments. For some individuals, watching and seeing racial trauma can merely be a nuisance. However, research suggests that for Black individuals, frequent exposure to the shootings of Black people can have long-term mental health effects. According to the psychologist Monnica Williams and colleagues (Malcoun et al., 2015), graphic videos combined with lived experiences of racism create severe psychological problems. The psychological symptoms are reminiscent of those associated with PTSD.

For the clinician, maintaining wellness is not just about keeping oneself well, it is also about the environment around them. This is particularly the case in racial trauma work, where systemic barriers or system failures can make it difficult for a practitioner to maintain wellness regardless of how much an individual tries. As does the total impact of racial trauma on our clients, systemic discrimination and related stressful events can have a cumulative impact on our effectiveness and how we function at work. Some of the barriers to wellness are based on the clinician's individual experiences and how those experiences affect them. Whether it is direct or indirect exposure to racial trauma, these experiences can make it difficult for a clinician to maintain their physical and emotional well-being.

Direct racially traumatic stressors include all direct traumatic contacts from living within a society of structural racism or being on the receiving end of individual racist attacks. A person experiencing a direct racial traumatic stressor may face microaggressions or macroassaults, barriers to employment, or harsh policing, or a host of inequitable policies throughout their daily life. The Black clinician is not immune to these stressors simply because they work in the mental health field. The Black clinician, in essence, finds themself in a double bind because not only do they experience racially traumatic events personally, they may also experience racially traumatic events vicariously through their clients.

There are two forms of vicarious racial traumatic stress for clinicians. The first can happen for any Black-identified individual: the stressful impact of living with systemic racism and witnessing other individuals contend with racial trauma. For example, watching the videos of unarmed Black individuals being killed by police, reading articles recounting the harmful treatment of Black individuals while partaking in everyday events (such as bird watching, shopping, or selling lemonade). The second is unique to Black clinicians. In addition to experiencing their own direct or vicarious racial trauma, the clinician will also have to hold space open for Black clients to process direct and vicarious trauma in an understanding environment. The strength this takes is not easy. Symptoms from experiencing racially traumatic events vicariously can mirror PTSD (intrusive symptoms, avoidance/numbing, negative thoughts/mood, hyperarousal/reactivity, and dissociative symptoms). However, symptoms unique to vicarious racial trauma are increased vigilance and suspicion, sensitivity to threat, psychological and physiological symptoms, alcohol and drug usage, and a narrowing sense of time (as listed and defined in Chapter 6).

Vicarious racial trauma exposure can severely affect how the clinician feels while doing this work and make the job feel much less enjoyable or productive than when they first began. In the case of Dr. Morris, there were many racially charged world events occurring back-to-back so quickly that she was unable to process her thoughts and feelings for herself before she was expected to work with her clients. Additionally, she was chosen because of her racial identity to counsel other Black-identified clients—far more than her peers were. What happened to Dr. Morris happens to many Black clinicians: Black clients want Black therapists, so the thinking is "Give them what they want." But, at what cost do we do that?

Where are all the Black clinicians? Nationally, 4% of psychologists (Hamp, Stamm, Lin, & Christidis, 2016); 2% of psychiatrists (Milloy, 2020); 22% of social workers (Pittman et al., 2021); 7% of marriage and family counselors; and 11% of professional counselors are reported to be Black. According to the 2022 Google trends data, the search term "Black therapist" rose substantially over the past 7 years, indicating an urgent and crucial demand for more Black clinicians. What should Morris's employer have done when the phone rang off the hook with Black clients asking to see a Black therapist? Here are a few ways Dr. Morris's employer could have responded.

- **Acknowledging the impact:** The supervisor could have started with a conversation with Dr. Morris. Beginning the conversation by acknowledging the racial trauma occurring during that time (and always) is impactful to the person experiencing the trauma. Dr. Morris may have finally felt seen by her employer for all of who she is, not just being a Black clinician who can help Black clients. Continuing the conversation by recognizing the impact that racial trauma is having on Dr. Morris is a key step. Acknowledging this impact opens the door for Dr. Morris to speak about the trauma's impact at work and with her supervisor. Ignoring this impact can lead to an employee or supervisee feeling shut down and not seen.

- **Acknowledging and addressing the situation:** Simply referring the majority of Black clients to Dr. Morris without a conversation as to why and recognizing the impact this may have on her were inevitably going to be detrimental. Discussing with the entire staff the shift in clientele, and brainstorming ways in which to tap into or even increase the competence of all clinicians working with Black-identified clients, would have been a valuable and important step. Rather than brushing racial topics under the rug, open dialogue makes it possible to discuss them in a constructive, helpful way. This openness allows clear communication about how best to support the clients and the staff.

- **Culturally responsive supervision:** While culturally responsive supervision should already be taking place (see Chapter 4), ensuring that it happens during critical times is imperative. Discussing with Dr. Morris her feelings about having more Black clients assigned to her, and what that might mean for her workload and for her mental health, would have been critical in the situation her agency was facing. Dr. Morris may very well have needed to take on more clients, and clients who are Black-identified, yet asking her to do so and not expecting the same from staff not identifying as Black are unfair. Additionally, it was important to determine what supports would have been helpful to put in place to buffer the effects of vicarious racial trauma.

Dr. Morris will also need to be an active participant in her healing from vicarious racial trauma. It is key that same-race and cross-racial clinicians understand the impact that racial trauma work will have on their own mental health. Vicarious racial trauma may result in their experiencing symptoms of anxiety, hypervigilance, poor concentration, or irritability. Vicarious racial traumatization can also have a deep impact on how the clinician understands themself and others. Monitor how experiences with racialized trauma can change the clinician's worldview.

According to Nancy Boyd-Franklin (Boyd-Franklin et al., 2015), therapists can engage in a host of activities to promote their **self-care**. Setting firm boundaries between work and home is a valuable coping strategy that helps to restore a sense of perspective and to maintain emotional stability. Additionally, taking care of oneself physically can add balance to life. Watching what one eats, getting enough rest and sleep, and even keeping physically active—all are useful forms of stress management and reduction. Even engaging in fun activities can lead to positive feelings and promote self-care. Laughter and humor can be tension releases, so watching a favorite TV show or a comedic film can lift a person's spirits and help them relax.

Psychological Health

Staying psychologically healthy means more than the counselor practicing simple self-care or avoiding racially traumatic stress when they can. Self-care to combat vicarious racial trauma must be an active process of maintaining wellness in all the areas of one's life. One of the benefits of addressing and maintaining wellness as a clinician is the greater likelihood that you will experience satisfaction at work and be less likely to burn out.

Burnout often reflects stress at the workplace that can lead to feeling overwhelmed and unhappy with the job. This experience is compounded for clinicians who identify with or relate to the victims of racially traumatic events. Experiences of vicarious racial trauma may make burnout happen more intensely and more quickly. When the clinician notices the first signs of burnout and vicarious racial trauma is when they should start thinking about how to get themselves back on track. The path to doing so is different for everyone, yet there are a few common steps.

- The counselor can consider which racially charged events have the greatest impact on them. Is it hearing personal stories from clients? Is it watching videos of people who share their identity being hurt, harmed, or killed? Or even experiencing one's own direct exposure to racially painful events? Knowing the answer will assist the counselor with clearly identifying that impact has occurred and they must take action.

- When thinking about the impact of vicarious racial trauma, it is important to notice some of the initial signs that cause one to become overwhelmed, indicating the impact of racial events. One of the signs Dr. Morris exhibited was a sense of helplessness while conducting therapy with people who were also Black and had experiences very similar to hers. That helplessness contributed to her feeling ineffective with her clients. She may have ignored this helpless feeling, which ultimately led to her leaving her counseling job. Experiences both within the counseling room and in the world can contribute to vicarious racial trauma and have a lasting impact if they go unaddressed.

- To combat racial vicarious trauma, the counselor can start by doing an inventory of how they care for themselves during some of the most difficult times. Caring for oneself can come in many different ways. The counselor might limit their intake of racially traumatic events by decreasing the amount of news and social media they consume. They should focus on bodily reactions and take the time needed to attend to the health of their body. For example, Dr. Morris was experiencing physical reactions such as headaches and she was emotionally exhausted every day. As her therapist, one could assist her with identifying the tools to manage her physical as well as psychological symptoms, like staying hydrated, walking, being connected to others, and so on. When a counselor's psychological self fails to tell them that they are not OK, sometimes their physical reactions can offer clues that they are not handling such stress well. Building skills to address symptoms allows for a set of tools that one can draw from, tools that have worked in the past during extremely painful events.

Most of the time we are not able to stop racial violence, mitigate microaggressions in the workplace, avoid the trauma our clients bring into the session, or a host of other issues that can add to our burnout.

This is why being intentional about self-care is crucial to prevent and buffer the effects of vicarious trauma and burnout. Using the tips above are just a start on the way to living a happier and healthier life.

Case Study: Shella

Shella is a 24-year-old Haitian female with a history of generalized anxiety disorder (GAD) who has been attending weekly therapy sessions for 8 weeks. Her therapist is Dr. Ingerson, a middle-aged white woman with 15 years of experience. Shella is a first-generation American, and her parents emigrated from Haiti before she was born. Shella lives with her parents, younger brother, paternal aunt, and maternal grandparents in the same home. Shella's family speaks Creole at home, and Shella's grandparents do not speak English. Shella's grandmother has been feeling sick with stomach pain for some time but refuses to go to the doctor despite Shella's encouraging. Therapy sessions have focused primarily on Shella's anxiety symptoms stemming from an unpleasant work environment and difficulty finding and keeping intimate relationships; however, Dr. Ingerson is aware of Shella's family dynamics from the intake session. Shella cancelled her last therapy session with Dr. Ingerson because of a family emergency. Shella presents for her ninth therapy session looking more distressed than usual.

DR. INGERSON: Hi, Shella, it's great to see you again. What would you like us to talk about today?

SHELLA: Last week, I had to rush my grandmother to the hospital because she was in so much pain. She kept saying she didn't want to go, but I took her anyway. After we got there and she was admitted, they did all of these tests on her. It turns out she has a big tumor in her stomach. She was in the hospital for a week.

DR. INGERSON: I'm so sorry to hear that. How are you handling all of this? [Here, the therapist reflected empathy and made room for Shella to express her emotions.]

SHELLA: Well, I stayed with her at the hospital, so I could translate for her what the doctors were saying, rather than waiting on the interpreter. That was exhausting. And I've been feeling really conflicted about some things lately.

DR. INGERSON: How so? [The therapist is probing for more, to really have Shella express the conflict she was feeling.]

SHELLA: At first, I was angry at her for refusing to go to the hospital. I thought if she had just gone when she first felt her pain, maybe this all could have been avoided. But, then when we were at the hospital, I could see why she resisted. I felt like the doctors didn't spend as much time with her because of all the translating. I could see the relief on their faces when they realized I spoke English. But, when I wasn't there, she didn't want to call for the nurse or ask for help. She was really in pain, but the doctors or nurses didn't take her seriously. It actually made me angry, especially when I realized this is why my Grann avoided the doctor . . . because she expected to be treated this way.

DR. INGERSON: How does it feel to say these concerns out loud to me? [Recognizing there are elements of culture and ethnicity embedded in Shella's recount, the therapist wisely paused to acknowledge that Shella is revealing all of this to a white therapist. This may have been hard for the therapist, but it was a necessary pause to acknowledge that it took courage for Shella to speak about her experience with racism, prejudice, and bias perpetrated by individuals who may look just like her therapist.]

SHELLA: I don't know . . . it's awkward, I guess. We haven't really talked about this kind of thing before. I don't want you to think that I mean all white doctors are bad.

The session continues with an honest, albeit uncomfortable and clunky, conversation about reconciling Shella's identities as both Haitian and American. Shella tiptoes around the subject of explicit racism, and Dr. Ingerson follows her lead and spends much of the session listening keenly. Afterward, Dr. Ingerson sits in her office and attempts to finish her notes, but she cannot shake a sense of inner emotional discord. "What kind of safe space am I creating if Shella is hesitant to talk about racism because I am white?," she thought. She recalled something her college-aged daughter mentioned to her about microaggressions: "What if I prove her right by inadvertently saying something offensive?"

Suddenly, her whiteness became the elephant in the room. To strengthen their therapeutic alliance, Dr. Ingerson decided to address it at the next session. She was no stranger to working through emotions that arise in the room, so why did this feel so daunting?

Race can feel like a taboo topic, even when it seems to be an obstacle to progress—especially for white therapists. Yet, leaving race out of the therapeutic discussion means Black clients will miss key support. Even before the kinds of violence, injuries, crimes, and cultural insults that prompted the BLM movement, white therapists were hesitant to raise issues of race with their Black clients. Counseling training programs that call for multicultural competency often fall short in many ways with educating therapists on how to truly relate and work with people of color. If the therapist is white, they may not have been taught how their own privilege reveals itself in a therapy setting. It is a privilege to not have to bring race into a therapeutic setting.

Elizabeth McCorvey (2020), a licensed clinical social worker, offered five ways in which a white therapist can engage clients through a more culturally informed lens. The first step is for the white therapist to build their skills by engaging in ongoing education on anti-racism and race. Attending trainings specifically on how to address race in the therapeutic setting and/or joining a peer supervision group with individuals who also want to learn and grow in this area is a great place to start. Additionally, obtaining a supervisor well versed in addressing race and issues around race in a therapeutic setting is also beneficial (though often hard to attain).

Second, a clinician can invite a discussion of race before the situation demands such conversation. In the case example above, Dr. Ingerson went nine sessions without opening the door to a conversation on race and the impact Shella's race may play on her presenting problems or impact the therapeutic relationship. During the intake sessions, Dr. Ingerson could have invited Shella to talk about how Dr. Ingerson's racial identity might influence their therapeutic relationship. For example, a question on the intake form should ask, "What it's like being a first-generation Haitian American?" Dr. Ingerson could have asked about any concerns or beliefs Shella may have had about the therapist's capacity to understand her experiences as a Black individual. Additionally in society, when a Black individual is hurt, harmed, or killed in a public manner because of their racial identity, a therapist may feel pressure to bring up the topic of race in the therapy space. However, if discussing issues of race and its impact on a client's reality is not a common conversation topic, the session can get awkward quickly. When the topic of race is a part of normal dialogue in sessions, there is an open invitation for these types of conversations to emerge. By laying a foundation where race is not a taboo topic, the door is open for the client to walk through it or just leave the door where it is.

The third suggestion is to engage in a discussion of race inside and outside of the therapy room. In the case of Dr. Ingerson, while writing her therapy notes, she contemplated whether she was creating a safe space if her client was hesitant to raise the topic of race. These thoughts would be wonderful to share with a peer support group or in supervision. The therapist should not experiment or practice having these conversations with the client. By practicing on a client, the client may end up feeling hurt by an insensitive remark, unaddressed microaggression, or ignorance. Having these conversations with friends, colleagues, and family is a great place to start when learning to sit with the discomfort that may arise when talking about racial topics.

Fourth, understand and know that it is OK to make mistakes. Dr. Ingerson was worried about saying something offensive to Shella; it is almost inevitable that therapists will make mistakes when discussing race and items of a sensitive nature. Acknowledging when mistakes are made and apologizing for them are a great place to start. To take it a step further, learn from the mistake and do things differently in the future. A strong therapeutic alliance can lend itself to an opportunity to repair the therapeutic relationship after a therapist does make a mistake.

Finally, the therapist may need to shift the way in which they view their Black clients. Instead of viewing Black clients as victims, think about how a particular individual faced great injustices throughout their life because of the color of their skin but still prevailed. Black clients are living in unjust systems that oppress and degrade them on a daily basis. Offering paths to healing, along with assisting clients to identify ways to navigate this world, can help them find concrete methods for contending with the systems that oppress them. Overall, a therapist without the lived experience of being Black in this world must recognize that there is a lot of work that needs to be done in systems, in those around them, and in themselves before any true healing can happen.

Psychologically Healthy Organizations

In the wake of consistent racial unrest and workplace racial microaggressions, often there are insufficient organizational strategies and resources to assist the Black counselor with resources to adapt to the increasing demands of their work. What can an organization do to assist their Black clinicians so they do not fall victim to the stressors and symptoms stemming from an unsupportive organization? First, acknowledge and accept that race is an organizing factor in society and in Black clinicians' lives. When an organization conveys a general understanding and acceptance of this premise, conversations and actions around race can occur. To do this, organizations need to be proactive, rather than reactive. Have a plan in place for Black clinicians when there is yet another national tragedy and Black clients seek treatment from Black practitioners. The plan can include limiting the number of specific types of clients a clinician may be assigned, assisting the clinician with integrating self-care throughout their day to help buffer the effects of vicarious racial trauma, and creating an avenue for culturally responsive supervision that is built into the job rather than only when tragedy strikes.

A clear feature of a responsive organization is allowing open discussions around race. This is important because an organization should not just talk about race when racial tragedy occurs, but always be actively engaged in such conversations around race and how one's race influences their work environment. To do this, the organization must actively create spaces where race can be discussed, examined, and celebrated. Below are four examples of ways in which organizations can be proactive.

1. **Equitable encounters:** Wanting to be proactive in their discussion about race in the workplace, companies can create so-called equitable encounters. Equitable encounters consist of small groups of 15–20 employees who voluntarily want to dive deeper into issues of race and diversity. This is a 90-minute session that is loosely structured around

current events related to race and diversity issues. These sessions can occur every 6–8 weeks, with the goal of these groups being a way to create a workspace that values and encourages such conversations.

2. **Diversity dives:** These sessions are companywide presentations on race, intersectionality, and diversity issues that give all employees the same information. They can be recorded for individuals who were not able to make the live sessions and would be required watching for them. The goal of these meetings is to allow all employees to learn through active listening without the pressure to discuss these issues if they are not ready to do so.

3. **P.E.A.C.E. (Positive Energy Activates Constant Elevation) groups:** This model is specifically intended for team meetings within a company that consist of 20–25 people per group. P.E.A.C.E. groups are topic-driven and structured around a specific topic, such as race; diversity, equity, inclusion (DEI); and access. One week before P.E.A.C.E. groups meet, an email should be distributed to participants asking them to read a particular article based on any number of topics, listen to a podcast about DEI, or watch culturally relevant videos. Having engaged in the same activity before the P.E.A.C.E. groups, the employees are then asked to come prepared to discuss the information as it relates to them, their work, and/or their understanding. The goal of these P.E.A.C.E. groups is to build a groundswell of positive energy around topics of race and diversity, which would, in turn, elevate employees' knowledge and understanding. Additionally, the size of these groups allows people who want to participate verbally to do just that, but there is no pressure for everyone to speak. All can learn!

4. **Management commitment sessions:** These sessions are created specifically for the leaders of an organization (the chief executive officer, chief operating officer, chief financial officer, upper-level management). These individuals can meet as a group to learn about the role of race-related issues: how they affect them, their employees, and the company. The group can also examine hiring practices, promotions, equity in pay, and more. The goals of these sessions are to assist upper-level management with continued growth in these areas as well as provide a space to

discuss the company's vision in the areas of diversity, justice, equity, and inclusion.

There are several ways an organization can help Black clinicians buffer the effects of racism and racial trauma. Please remember that an *organization* is not just a building or an address, but rather all the people who make up that organization. A critical piece of building organizational support for Black clinicians is fostering cultural humility among coworkers, fostering an eagerness to learn about the organizing principle of race, and building a sense of community. To the degree possible, all employees should be engaged in a discussion that leads to understanding and clear communication around racial issues.

Counselors or consultants should continue to work on reducing their discomfort with racial topics. The key is to know, understand, and talk about the importance of culture and recent events with all clients and consultees, regardless of race. For example, a therapist should talk to all of their clients about current events when race-related stories dominate the media no matter the client's race. The more one does this, the more comfortable they become.

CHAPTER TAKEAWAYS

- Any clinician should not attempt to process racially charged situations in the media with clients before they have processed those same situations with themself. This may be hard to do when a racialized event occurs every second of every day. However, the counselor should do what they can to process the parts of a story that bother them the most with their colleagues and peers before they address it with clients.

- Particularly important in cross-racial situations, try not to personalize the client's response or anger. Remember, this is not about the counselor but about the client's experience of racism.

- The counselor can become a part of a peer consultation group where they feel comfortable, processing racially charged events that may come up in the therapeutic process with their clients.

- Organizational issues can have a severe individual impact on Black clinicians dealing with racism and varying forms of racial trauma. An example would be depression, where the counselor may feel as if they do not have the energy to accomplish everything that needs to be done at work. This can lead to unproductive thoughts and wondering whether what they are doing constitutes worthwhile work. To combat such a mindset, the organization must be proactive rather than reactive when examining, addressing, and celebrating race.

- The counselor needs to remind themself of those areas where they do have control. It is not the counselor's job to get rid of systemic racism! The key takeaway is to find the locus of control. Then make space for clients and organizations to process and provide supports to themselves or their employees. This is how we slowly dismantle systemic racism and the structures that keep it in place.

Conclusion
Summing It All Up

We close the book by revisiting some of the key themes we have discussed.

Recall the comment from the African American client mentioned in Chapter 1: "I stay ready, so I don't have to get ready." What is the toll of living under constant threat? The traumas of chronic stress and racism are inextricably linked. Racial trauma is the occurrence of any racialized event or experience that renders a person powerless over their own physical integrity, with a feeling of hopelessness and a foreshortened future. Hopelessness results in feelings of significant vulnerability and inability to cope with racial trauma reminders and stressors. Racial trauma changes the way people move in the world and, consequently, how that impacts relationships. The discussions, ideas, and examples in this book were geared to create a more culturally responsive, trauma-informed clinician. And that means the clinician needs to understand racial trauma: how it shows up in those served, in those supervised, and within themself.

Woven within the chapters are the experiences of Black individuals who remain underrepresented in the development of Eurocentric treatments and diagnoses. This is not to say that these treatments do not work with Black individuals, as we know these treatments can be widely effective with diverse populations. But when treatments do not work, what other options do we have? This book explored the most prominent examples of diagnostic and treatment trends that result in poor outcomes for Black people and offered concrete suggestions for improving outcomes and treatment seeking.

For Black individuals, finding a clinician who is culturally humble, willing to learn, and ready to apply that knowledge is often hard. Black clients often drop out of therapy because they encounter therapists who have not done their own introspective work around race and its impact on Black clients, or therapists who use strictly Eurocentric frameworks to fix a problem, rather than explore healing or soul care. The fit between the clinician and the Black individual seeking help is identified as being one of the most important predictors of that client's outcome. Clinicians should work together through peer supervision, joining state and national professional associations, and engaging in continuing education to promote culturally responsive treatment.

In this book, we delved into a variety of contexts and systems in which clinicians encounter racial trauma. The school-to-prison pipeline is real! Clinicians working in school systems can educate, advocate, and intervene in a meaningful way that can disrupt the effects of racial trauma. School clinicians should take active roles to influence policies that directly or indirectly target Black students negatively. In addition, clinicians should critically examine the influence that racial trauma has on potential achievement gaps and discipline practices in their school. It may be hard for a clinician to recognize the influence they hold in their school. However, once that influence is recognized, there is power in the clinician's voice and actions. School clinicians should never resign themselves to the idea that their school system cannot change. Change comes with action and follow-up.

Clinicians working with Black individuals employed by law enforcement agencies are in a unique position to examine racial trauma from two perspectives. The first perspective is that of a professional working in a system that was built on institutionalized racism. The second is that of individuals within the system who have faced racial trauma themselves. Clinicians working with Black law enforcement officers need to maintain a delicate balance between those individuals' two identities. The clinician's role is to assist such individuals with racial trauma in an open, factual, and compassionate way. This may feel like a heavy lift, but if clinicians who do this work continue to engage in their own work, it will alleviate some of their own anxiety around race, institutional racism, and racial traumatic stress. This ongoing training and personal work will then assist the clinician in addressing the needs of Black officers.

Working with Black parents and families gives practitioners a unique opportunity to understand how parents engage in the racial socialization of their children to help them navigate the world. The clinician should take the time to understand some common Black family dynamics and the impact on child-rearing of living in a country that was built on racism. Every time the story of a young Black child being hurt, harmed, or killed surfaces, there is a sense of fear and anger, and reinforcement of the duty that Black parents have internalized: They must do everything in their power to make sure their children are safe in a world that still sees them as dangerous.

When working with Black clients who have faced racially charged events, clinicians sometimes jump to the conclusion that it is their job to address such a situation and fix it. But as we have discussed, there is another more holistic way of working with Black clients, and that is not to "fix" anything, but to *assist* the client with healing from the impact of these experiences. One does not simply "get over" a racially traumatic experience. But clinicians can help by acknowledging, believing, and affirming that a client's trauma is real, does exist. Clinicians should work hard to create a language for the experiences that Black clients contend with in a world full of racism. Having that language enables the clinician to assist Black clients with naming their experiences. Naming the experiences is the beginning of healing from them.

Black clinicians working with Black clients may have racial experiences in common with their clients, which can affect the clinician's sense of self and well-being. Cross-racial clinicians can also feel the impact and pain of their clients and that can overly impact their own well-being. In the same way that racial trauma has a cumulative impact on clients, racial trauma and related stressful events can have a cumulative impact on the clinician, impacting their effectiveness at work. Whether they are directly exposed to racial trauma or more indirect forms, these experiences can make it difficult for a clinician to maintain their physical, emotional, and other forms of wellness. On-the-job stressors along with the injustice ongoing around them can lead practitioners to experience burnout. Clinicians need to devote time to keeping themselves well, but it is also vital to create a supportive environment around them to help sustain their wellness. This is particularly the case in racial trauma work where systemic barriers or systems failures can undermine efforts to maintain wellness.

In sum, the sensitive and prepared clinician can have a healing impact on the lives of Black clients from varying backgrounds, from parents, to students, to officers, and to supervisees. There may be feelings of awkwardness that come when implementing the techniques in this book with Black clients who have experienced racial trauma. There may be fear of causing more harm, making mistakes, or even offending someone when addressing traumatic stress symptoms. However, everyone "messes up" from time to time. Clinicians do not always get it right, and that's OK! The key is to keep learning and to not be afraid to apply this newly learned knowledge with your clients. This is not easy work. However, it is work that is worth learning and doing because of the impact it will have on the well-being of Black clients.

Glossary

Achievement gap—The disparities in educational achievement between different racial groups.

African/Black psychology—According to the Association of Black Psychologists, "a dynamic manifestation of unifying African principles, values and traditions. It is the self-conscious 'centering' of psychological analyses and applications in African realities, cultures, and epistemologies. Black/African centered psychology, as a system of thought and action, examines the processes that allow for the illumination and liberation of the Spirit. Relying on the principles of harmony within the universe as a natural order of existence, Black/African centered psychology recognizes: the Spirit that permeates everything that is; the notion that everything in the universe is interconnected; the value that the collective is the most salient element of existence; and the idea that communal self-knowledge is the key to mental health. Black/African centered psychology is ultimately concerned with understanding the systems of meaning of human beingness, the features of human functioning, and the restoration of normal/natural order to human development. As such, it is used to resolve personal and social problems and to promote optimal functioning" (Association of Black Psychologists, 2022, p. 1).

Black Lives Matter (BLM)—An international activist movement, originating in the African American community, that campaigns against violence and systemic racism toward Black people. BLM regularly protests police killings of Black people and broader issues of racial profiling, police brutality, and racial inequality in the U.S. criminal justice system.

Blue Lives Matter—A countermovement in the United States that emerged in 2014 in direct opposition to the Black Lives Matter movement. A group of law enforcement officers, both active and retired, formed Blue Lives Matter to challenge media reports that they perceived to be anti-police.

Burnout—According to WebMD, a form of exhaustion caused by constantly feeling swamped. It happens when we experience too much emotional, physical, and mental fatigue for too long. In many cases, burnout is related to one's job. But burnout can also happen in other areas of your life and affect your health.

Called in—The act of checking the actions of your peers and getting them to change problematic behaviors by explaining their missteps with compassion and patience.

Called out—A public immediate action, always appropriate, to stop words or actions that are actively hurting someone. It may be reactive to disrupt discriminatory behavior.

Civil rights—The rights of citizens to political and social freedom and equality. The civil rights movement was a struggle for justice and equality for African Americans that took place mainly in the 1950s and 1960s.

Code switching—Changing one's speech, appearance, or behavior to fit in and to put others at ease.

Complex trauma—Describes exposure to multiple traumatic events—often of an invasive, interpersonal nature—and the wide-ranging, long-term effects of this exposure. These events are severe and pervasive, such as abuse or profound neglect.

Creating a Respectful and Open World for Natural Hair (CROWN) Act—In 2019, the bill was introduced in the U. S. Congress. It was intended to prohibit discrimination based on an individual's hair texture or hairstyle by classifying such discrimination as illegal under federal law.

Cultural competence—Behaviors, attitudes, and policies that, when taken together, work to ensure that systems and people within those systems can engage with diverse cultural groups appropriately and in an efficient manner.

Cultural humility—The ability to maintain an interpersonal stance of openness to another regarding aspects of cultural identities.

Discrimination—The unfair or prejudicial treatment of people and groups based on characteristics such as race, gender, national origin.

Equity—Refers to fairness and justice and is distinguished from equality. Whereas equality means providing the same to all, equity means recognizing that we do not all start from the same place and must acknowledge and make adjustments to imbalances. The process is ongoing, requiring us to identify and overcome intentional and unintentional barriers arising from bias or systemic structures.

Explicit bias—The traditional conceptualization of bias. With explicit bias, individuals are aware of their prejudices and attitudes toward certain groups. Overt racism and racist comments are examples of explicit biases.

Hidden spot—Indication that people may be unaware of their implicit biases or ignorance of certain cultural norms different than their own.

Implicit bias—Includes the subconscious feelings, attitudes, prejudices, and stereotypes an individual has developed due to prior influences and imprints throughout their lives. Individuals are unaware that subconscious perceptions, instead of facts and observations, affect their decision making.

Internalized racism—Occurs when a person accepts negative stereotypes of an oppressed/marginalized group of which they are a member. This emotional and cognitive acceptance of such stereotypes can result in shame, guilt, and anger that may be demonstrated by rejecting the people, images, and markers of their own culture. It might result in efforts to deny being a part of that culture or trying to create distance in some way from being associated with it.

Macroassaults—Large-scale or overt aggression toward those of a certain race, culture, gender, or another characteristic. Macroaggressions affect whole classes of groups of populations and reside in the structures, programs, policies of institutions, society, and our customs.

Microaggressions—A comment or action that subtly and often unconsciously or unintentionally expresses a prejudiced attitude toward a member of a marginalized group.

Motivational interviewing (MI)—A guiding style of communication that sits between good listening and giving information and advice. It is designed to empower people to change by drawing out their own meaning, importance, and capacity for change. It is also based on a respectful and curious way of being with people that facilitates the natural process of change and honors client autonomy (Miller & Rollnick, 2012).

Posttraumatic stress disorder (PTSD)—A psychiatric disorder that may occur in people who have experienced or witnessed a traumatic event, series of events, or set of circumstances. An individual may experience this as emotionally or physically harmful or life-threatening, and it may affect mental, physical, social, and/or spiritual well-being.

Privilege—A special right, advantage, or immunity granted or available only to a particular person or group.

Psychological trauma—A person's experience of emotional distress resulting from an event that overwhelms the capacity to emotionally digest it. The precipitating event may be a one-time occurrence or a series of occurrences perceived as seriously harmful or life- threatening to oneself or loved ones.

Race-based traumatic stress—Speaks to the unique psychological and emotional distress that Black, Indigenous, and People of Color (BIPOC) suffer because of racism and discrimination. These experiences can occur on a macro, meso, or micro level.

Racial identity—A sense of self that is linked to membership in a racial group. This includes more than physical attributes, but also other relevant aspects of attitudes and behaviors affiliated with that racial group.

Racial oppression—Burdening a specific race with unjust or cruel restraints or impositions. Racial oppression may be social, systematic, institutionalized, or internalized.

Racial trauma—The stressful impact or emotional pain of one's experience with racism, discrimination, and racial violence.

Racism—The systemic oppression of a racial group to the social, economic, and political advantage of another.

Reflective local practice (RLP)—An approach to mental health work that includes reflecting on the culture and climate of the community and organizations in which the mental health provider serves. It intends for the practitioner to engage in this reflection as a method of providing services in a way that is attuned to the needs and culture of the community.

School-to-prison pipeline—A nationwide system of local, state, and federal education and public safety policies that pushes students out of school and into the criminal justice system. The system disproportionately targets youth of color and youth with disabilities.

Self-care—The practice of taking an active role in protecting one's own well-being and happiness, in particular during periods of stress.

Stigmatization—The action of describing or regarding someone or something as worthy of disgrace or great disapproval.

Structural racism—Refers to the totality of ways in which societies foster racial discrimination through mutually reinforcing systems of housing, education, employment, earnings, benefits, credit, media, health care, and criminal justice. These patterns and practices, in turn, reinforce discriminatory beliefs, values, and distribution of resources.

Toxic stress—This is the body's response to lasting and serious stress, without enough support from others. When a person doesn't get the help they need, their body cannot turn off the stress response normally. This lasting stress can harm the body and brain of a person and cause lifelong health problems.

Trauma—When a person experiences very stressful, frightening, or distressing events that are difficult to cope with or out of their control. It could be one incident, or an ongoing event that happens over a long period of time.

Vicarious racial trauma—The secondhand exposure to racial trauma, discrimination, and/or prejudice directed at another individual. In order for an exposure to racial trauma to be considered vicarious, the unintended victim must be cognizant of someone else experiencing racial trauma.

Vicarious trauma—An ongoing process of change over time that results from witnessing or hearing about other people's suffering and need.

References

Alexander K. L., Entwisle D. R., & Thompson M. S. (1987). School performance, status relations, and the structure of sentiment: Bringing the teacher back in. *American Sociological Review, 52*, 665–682.

American Civil Liberties Union. (2022). What is the school-to-prison pipeline? *www.aclu.org/documents/what-school-prison-pipeline*

American Psychological Association. (2014). Guidelines for clinical Supervision in health service psychology. *http://apa.org/about/policy/guidelines-supervision.pdf*

American Psychological Association. (2022). Demographics of U.S. psychology workforce [Interactive data tool]. *www.apa.org/workforce/data-tools/demographics*

American School Counselor Association. (2021). The school counselor and cultural diversity. *www.schoolcounselor.org/Standards-Positions/Position-Statements/ASCA-Position-Statements/The-School-Counselor-and-Cultural-Diversity*

Anderson, R. E., Jones, S. C., Saleem, F. T., Metzger, I., Anyiwo, N., Nisbeth, K. S., . . . Stevenson, H. C. (2021). Interrupting the pathway from discrimination to African American adolescents' psychosocial outcomes: The contribution of parental racial worries and racial socialization competency. *Child Development, 92*(6), 2375–2394.

Anderson, R. E., Jones, S. C., & Stevenson, H. C. (2020). The initial development and validation of the Racial Socialization Competency Scale: Quality and quantity. *Cultural Diversity and Ethnic Minority Psychology, 26*(4), 426.

Anderson, R. E., McKenny, M. C., & Stevenson, H. C. (2019). EMBRace: Developing a racial socialization intervention to reduce racial stress and enhance racial coping among Black parents and adolescents. *Family Process, 58*(1), 53–67.

Anderson, M. (2016). How the stress of racism affects learning. *The Atlantic*.

Angelou, M. (1997). *I know why the caged bird sings*. Bantam.

Arredondo, P. (2019). *Eliminating race-based mental health disparities: Promoting equity and culturally responsive care across settings*. New Harbinger Publications.

Ashley, W., & Lipscomb, A. E. (2018). Culturally affirming clinical supervision in graduate field education: Enhancing transformative dialogue in the supervisory dyad. *International Research in Higher Education, 3*(3), 22

Assari, S. (2019). Parental educational attainment and academic performance of American college students; Blacks' diminished returns. *Journal of Health Economics and Development, 1*(1), 21.

Assari, S., Mardani, A., Maleki, M., Boyce, S., & Bazargan, M. (2021). Black–White achievement gap: Role of race, school urbanity, and parental education. *Pediatric Health, Medicine and Therapeutics, 12*, 1–11.

Association of Black Psychologists. (2022). The Black Mental Health Workforce Survey Report. chrome-extension://efaidnbmnnnibpcajpcglclefindmkaj/https://abpsi.org/wp-content/uploads/2022/12/The-Black-Mental-Health-Workforce-Survey-Final.pdf

Auguste, E., Lodge, T., Carrenard, N., Onwong'a, J. R., Zollicoffer, A., Collins, D., & London, L. (2024). Seeing one another: The creation of the Sawubona healing circles. *Journal of Black Psychology, 50*(4), 411–447.

Ayalon, L., & Alvidrez, J. (2007). The experience of black consumers in the mental health system—Identifying barriers to and facilitators of mental health treatment using the consumers' perspective. *Issues in Mental Health Nursing, 28*(12), 1323–1340.

Baier, A. L., Kline, A. C., & Feeny, N. C. (2020). Therapeutic alliance as a mediator of change: A systematic review and evaluation of research. *Clinical Psychology Review, 82*, 101921.

Baldwin, J., Capouya, E., Hansberry, L, Hentoff, N., Hughes, L., & Kazin, A. (1961). The Negro in American culture. *CrossCurrents, 11*(3), 205–225.

Barnes, A. (2008). Race and hospital diagnoses of schizophrenia and mood disorders. *Social Work, 53*(1), 77–83.

Bates, B. R., & Harris, T. M. (2004). The Tuskegee Study of Untreated Syphilis and public perceptions of biomedical research: A focus group study. *Journal of the National Medical Association, 96*(8), 1051.

Beck, A. T., Epstein, N., Brown, G., & Steer, R. A. (1988). An inventory for measuring clinical anxiety: Psychometric properties. *Journal of Consulting and Clinical Psychology, 56*(6), 893.

Beck, J. S., & Wright, J. H. (1997). Cognitive therapy: Basics and beyond. *Journal of Psychotherapy Practice and Research, 6,* 71–80.

Blaustein, M. E., & Kinniburgh, K. M. (2018). *Treating traumatic stress in children and adolescents: How to foster resilience through attachment, self-regulation, and competency.* Guilford Press.

Boyd-Franklin, N. (2013). *Black families in therapy: Understanding the African American experience.* Guilford Press.

Boyd-Franklin, N., Cleek, E. N., Wofsy, M., & Mundy, B. (2015). *Therapy in the real world: Effective treatments for challenging problems.* Guilford Press.

Bradley, K. (2022). The socioeconomic achievement gap in the U.S. public schools. *Ballard Brief, 2022*(3), 10.

Burkard, A. W., Johnson, A. J., Madson, M. B., Pruitt, N. T., Contreras-Tadych, D. A., Kozlowski, J. M., . . . Knox, S. (2006). Supervisor cultural responsiveness and unresponsiveness in cross-cultural supervision. *Journal of Counseling Psychology, 53*(3), 288.

Cabral, R., & Smith, T. B. (2011). Racial/ethnic matching of clients and therapists in mental health services: A meta-analytic review of preferences, perceptions, and outcomes. *Journal of Counseling Psychology, 58,* 537–554.

Calloway, A., & Creed, T. A. (2022). Enhancing CBT consultation with multicultural counseling principles. *Cognitive and Behavioral Practice, 29*(4), 787–795.

Cokley, K., & Garba, R. (2018). Speaking truth to power: How Black/African psychology changed the discipline of psychology. *Journal of Black Psychology, 44*(8), 695–721.

Constantine, M. G., & Sue, D. W. (2007). Perceptions of racial microaggressions among black supervisees in cross-racial dyads. *Journal of Counseling Psychology, 54*(2), 142.

Cronholm, P. F., Forke, C. M., Wade, R., Bair-Merritt, M. H., Davis, M., Harkins-Schwarz, . . . Fein, J. A. (2015). Adverse childhood experiences: Expanding the concept of adversity. *American Journal of Preventive Medicine, 49*(3), 354–361.

Davis, A. Y. (2003). *Are prisons obsolete?* Seven Stories Press.

DeAngelis, T. (2015, March 1). In search of cultural competence. *Monitor on Psychology, 46*(3), 64.

DeGruy-Leary, J. (2017). *Post-traumatic slave syndrome: America's legacy of enduring injury.* Joy DeGruy.

Dye, H. (2018). The impact and long-term effects of childhood trauma. *Journal of Human Behavior in the Social Environment, 28*(3), 381–392.

El-Mekki, S. (2021). Most white teachers are not ready to teach black and brown students. *www.edpost.com/stories/most-white-teachers-are-not-ready-to-teach-black-and-brown-students*

Falender, C. A., & Shafranske, E. P. (2021). *Clinical supervision: A competency-based approach* (2nd ed.). American Psychological Association.

Falender, C. A., Shafranske, E. P., & Falicov, C. J. (2014). *Multiculturalism and diversity in clinical supervision: A competency-based approach* (pp. xv–296). American Psychological Association.

Felitti, V. J., Anda, R. F., Nordenberg, D., Williamson, D. F., Spitz, A. M., Edwards, V., & Marks, J. S. (1998). Relationship of childhood abuse and household dysfunction to many of the leading causes of death in adults: The Adverse Childhood Experiences (ACE) Study. *American Journal of Preventive Medicine, 14*(4), 245–258.

Ferguson R. F. (2003). Teachers' perceptions and expectations and the Black–White test score gap. *Urban Education, 38*, 460–507.

Fisher, B. W., & Devlin, D. N. (2024). Cops and counselors: How school staffing decisions relate to exclusionary discipline rates and racial/ethnic disparities. *Race and Social Problems, 16*(1), 19–46.

Ford, J. D., Stockton, P., Kaltman, S., & Green, B. L. (2006). Disorders of extreme stress (DESNOS) symptoms are associated with type and severity of interpersonal trauma exposure in a sample of healthy young women. *Journal of Interpersonal Violence, 21*(11), 1399–1416.

Fukuyama, M. A. (1994). Critical incidents in multicultural counseling supervision: A phenomenological approach to supervision research. *Counselor Education and Supervision, 34*(2), 142–151.

Gara, M. A., Minsky, S., Silverstein, S. M., Miskimen, T., & Strakowski, S. M. (2019). A naturalistic study of racial disparities in diagnoses at an outpatient behavioral health clinic. *Psychiatric Services, 70*(2), 130–134.

García, E. (2020). *Schools are still segregated, and Black children are paying a price*. Economic Policy Institute.

Gibbs, T. A., Okuda, M., Oquendo, M. A., Lawson, W. B., Wang, S., Thomas, Y. F., & Blanco, C. (2013). Mental health of African Americans and Caribbean blacks in the United States: Results from the national epidemiological survey on alcohol and related conditions. *American Journal of Public Health, 103*(2), 330–338.

Gladwell, M. (2019). *Talking to strangers: What we should know about the people we don't know*. Little, Brown.

Greene-Moton, E., & Minkler, M. (2020). Cultural competence or cultural humility? Moving beyond the debate. *Health Promotion Practice, 21*(1), 142–145.

Gregory, A., Skiba, R. J., & Noguera, P. A. (2010). The achievement gap and the discipline gap: Two sides of the same coin? *Educational Researcher, 39*, 59–68.

Gregory, A., & Weinstein, R. (2008). The discipline gap and African Americans: Defiance or cooperation in the classroom. *Journal of School Psychology, 46*(4), 455–475.

Grills, C., & Ajei, M. (2002). African-centered conceptualizations of self and consciousness: The Akan model. In T. A. Parham (Ed.), *Counseling persons of African descent: Raising the bar of practitioner competence* (pp. 75–99). Sage.

Guthrie, R. V. (2004). *Even the rat was white: A historical view of psychology.* Pearson Education.

Hamp, A., Stamm, K., Lin, L., & Christidis, P. (2016). *2015 APA survey of psychology health service providers.* American Psychological Association.

Hardy, K. V. (2013). Healing the hidden wounds of racial trauma. *Reclaiming Children and Youth, 22*(1), 24.

Hardy, K. V. (2023). *Racial trauma: Clinical strategies and techniques for healing invisible wounds.* Norton.

Harris, N. B. (2018). *The deepest well: Healing the long-term effects of childhood adversity.* Houghton Mifflin Harcourt.

Hays, P. A. (2001). *Addressing cultural complexities in practice: A framework for clinicians and counselors* (pp. 3–16). Washington, DC: American Psychological Association.

Henderson, R. C., Williams, P., Gabbidon, J., Farrelly, S., Schauman, O., Hatch, S., & MIRIAD Study Group. (2015). Mistrust of mental health services: Ethnicity, hospital admission and unfair treatment. *Epidemiology and Psychiatric Sciences, 24*(3), 258–265.

Hines, P. M., Macias, C., & Perrino, T. (2014). Implementing a violence intervention for inner-city adolescents: Potential pitfalls and suggested remedies. In J. A. Durlak & J. R. Ferrari (Eds.), *Program implementation in preventive trials* (pp. 35–49). Routledge.

Hoffman, K. M., Trawalter, S., Axt, J. R., & Oliver, M. N. (2016). Racial bias in pain assessment and treatment recommendations, and false beliefs about biological differences between blacks and whites. *Proceedings of the National Academy of Sciences, 113*(16), 4296–4301.

Hohman, M. (2021). *Motivational interviewing in social work practice.* Guilford Press.

Hook, J. N., Davis, D. E., Owen, J., Worthington, Jr., E. L., & Utsey, S. O. (2013). Cultural humility: Measuring openness to culturally diverse clients. *Journal of Counseling Psychology, 60*(3), 353.

Howard, G. R. (2016). *We can't teach what we don't know: White teachers, multiracial schools*. Teachers College Press.

Huang, F. L., & Cornell, D. G. (2017). Student attitudes and behaviors as explanations for the Black–White suspension gap. *Children and Youth Services Review, 73*, 298–308.

Jacobsen, W., Pace, G., & Rmirez, N., (2019). Punishment and inequality at an early age: Exclusionary discipline in elementary school. *Social Forces, 97*(3).

Jones, J. R., & Gregory, A. (2011). Examining the relationship between school discipline and dropout for Black students. *The PsychDiscourse, 45*, 3.

Jones, N., Marks, N., Ramirez, R., & Rios-Vargas, M. (2021, August 12). 2020 Census illuminates racial and ethnic composition of the country. United States Census Bureau. *www.census.gov/library/stories/2021/08/improved-race-ethnicity-measures-reveal-united-states-population-much-more-multiracial.html*

Jones, S. C., Anderson, R. E., & Stevenson, H. C. (2021). Not the same old song and dance: Viewing racial socialization through a family systems lens to resist racial trauma. *Adversity and Resilience Science, 2*, 225–233.

Kidane, S., & Rauscher, E. (2023). Unequal exposure to school resource officers, by student race, ethnicity, and income. Urban Institute. *www.urban.org/sites/default/files/2023-04/Unequal%20Exposure%20to%20School%20Resource%20Officers%2C%20by%20Student%20Race%2C%20Ethnicity%2C%20and%20Income.pdf*

Levy, D. J., Heissel, J. A., Richeson, J. A., & Adam, E. K. (2016). Psychological and biological responses to race-based social stress as pathways to disparities in educational outcomes. *American Psychologist, 71*(6), 455.

Leiber, M. J., & Fix, R. (2019). Reflections on the impact of race and ethnicity on juvenile court outcomes and efforts to enact change. *American Journal of Criminal Justice, 44*, 581–608.

Long, D. A., McCoach, D. B., Siegle, D., Callahan, C. M., & Gubbins, E. J. (2023). Inequality at the starting line: Underrepresentation in gifted identification and disparities in early achievement. *AERA Open, 9*, 23328584231171535.

Malcoun, E., Williams, M. T., & Nouri, L. B. (2015). Assessment of posttraumatic stress disorder with African Americans. In L. T. Benuto & B. D. Leany (Eds.), *Guide to Psychological Assessment with African Americans* (pp. 163–182). Springer Science + Business Media.

Mann, A., Whitaker, A., Torres-Gullien, S., Morton, M., Jordan, H., Coyle, S., & Sun, W. L. (2019). Cops and no counselors: How the lack of school mental health staff is harming students. *www.aclu.org/wp-content/uploads/publications/030419-acluschooldisciplinereport.pdf*

McCarter, S., Venkitasubramanian, K., & Bradshaw, K. (2019). Addressing the school-to-prison pipeline: Examining micro-and macro-level variables that affect school disengagement and subsequent felonies. *Journal of Social Service Research, 46*(3), 379–393.

McCorvey, E. (2020). *Stop hesitating: A resource for psychotherapists and counselors*. ACPE News.

Merolla, D. M., & Jackson, O. (2019). Structural racism as the fundamental cause of the academic achievement gap. *Sociology Compass, 13*(6), e12696.

Merriam-Webster. (2023). Mediation. www.merriam-webster.com/dictionary/mediation

Metzger, I. W., Anderson, R. E., Are, F., & Ritchwood, T. (2021). Healing interpersonal and racial trauma: Integrating racial socialization into trauma-focused cognitive behavioral therapy for African American youth. *Child Maltreatment, 26*(1), 17–27.

Michael, A. (2015). *Raising race questions: Whiteness and inquiry in education*. Teachers College Press.

Miller, W. R., & Rollnick, S. (2012). *Motivational interviewing: Helping people change*. Guilford press.

Milloy, C. (2020). Black psychiatrists are few. They've never been more needed. *Washington Post, 11*.

Monahan, K. C., VanDerhei, S., Bechtold, J., & Cauffman, E. (2014). From the school yard to the squad car: School discipline, truancy, and arrest. *Journal of Youth and Adolescence, 43*, 1110–1122.

Morgan, P. L., Wang, Y., Woods, A. D., Mandel, Z., Farkas, G., & Hillemeier, M. M. (2019). Are U.S. schools discriminating when suspending students with disabilities? A best-evidence synthesis. *Exceptional Children, 86*(1), 7–24.

Morrison, T. (1987). *Beloved/Toni Morrison*. Alfred A. Knopf.

Myles, T. L. (2020). The silent disease of law enforcement officers: The stigma of mental health in law enforcement identity and mental health outcomes. *Doctoral Dissertations and Projects, 2545*. https://digitalcommons.liberty.edu/doctoral/2545

National Center for Education Statistics. (2023). Characteristics of public school teachers. *Condition of Education*. U.S. Department of Education, Institute of Education Sciences. https://nces.ed.gov/programs/coe/indicator/clr

National Center for Education Statistics. (2024). Achievement gaps. U.S. Department of Education, Institute of Education Sciences. https://nces.ed.gov/nationsreportcard/studies/gaps/#:~:text=Achievement%20gaps%20occur%20when%20one,than%20the%20margin%20of%20error

National Child Traumatic Stress Network, Justice Consortium, Schools

Committee, and Culture Consortium. (2017). *Addressing race and trauma in the classroom: A resource for educators*. National Center for Child Traumatic Stress.

Neblett, E. W., Jr., White, R. L., Ford, K. R., Philip, C. L., Nguyen, H. X., & Sellers, R. M. (2008). Patterns of racial socialization and psychological adjustment: Can parental communications about race reduce the impact of racial discrimination? *Journal of Research on Adolescence, 18*(3), 477–515.

Nelson, L., & Lind, D. (2015, October 27). The school-to-prison pipeline explained. *Vox.* www.vox.com/2015/2/24/8101289/school-discipline-race

Nowicki, J. (2018). *Discipline disparities for Black students, boys, and students with disabilities* (Report No. GAO-18-258). Government Accountability Office.

Nowicki, J. M. (2022). *K–12 education: Student population has significantly diversified, but many schools remain divided along racial, ethnic, and economic lines*. Committee on Education and Labor, House of Representatives (Report No. GAO-22-104737). Government Accountability Office.

Office of Juvenile Justice and Delinquency Prevention. (2022, March). Racial and ethnic disparity in juvenile justice processing. https://ojjdp.ojp.gov/model-programs-guide/literature-reviews/racial-and-ethnic-disparity

Okonofua, J. A., Walton, G. M., & Eberhardt, J. L. (2016). A vicious cycle: A social–psychological account of extreme racial disparities in school discipline. *Perspectives on Psychological Science, 11*(3), 381–398.

Oluo, I. (2019). *So you want to talk about race*. Hachette UK.

Parker, J. S., Purvis, L., & Williams, B. (2023). Religious/spiritual struggles and mental health among black adolescents and emerging adults: A metasynthesis. *Journal of Black Psychology, 49*(2), 153–199.

Pittman, P., Chen, C., Erikson, C., Salsberg, E., Luo, Q., Vichare, A., . . . Burke, G. (2021). Health workforce for health equity. *Medical Care, 59*, S405–S408.

Pope, C. E., & Feyerherm, W. (1990). Minority status and juvenile justice processing. *Criminal Justice Abstracts, 22*(2), 327–336 (part 1); 22(3), 527–542 (part 2).

Pope, C. E., Lovell, R., & Hsia, H. M. (2002). *Disproportionate minority confinement: A review of the research literature from 1989 through 2001*. Bulletin. Office of Juvenile Justice and Delinquency Prevention, U.S. Department of Justice.

Prison Policy Initiative COVID-19 resources. (2023). COVID-19 in prisons and jails. *www.prisonpolicy.org/virus.*

Puzzanchera, C., Sladky, A. & Kang, W. (2020). Easy access to juvenile populations: 1990–2019. National Center for Juvenile Justice. www.ojjdp.gov/ojstatbb/ezapop

Roberts, A. L., Gilman, S. E., Breslau, J., Breslau, N., & Koenen, K. C. (2011). Race/ethnic differences in exposure to traumatic events, development of post-traumatic stress disorder, and treatment-seeking for post-traumatic stress disorder in the United States. *Psychological Medicine, 41*(1), 71–83.

Romijn, B. R., Slot, P. L., & Leseman, P. P. (2021). Increasing teachers' intercultural competences in teacher preparation programs and through professional development: A review. *Teaching and Teacher Education, 98*, 103236.

Sandeen, E., Moore, K. M., & Swanda, R. M. (2018). Reflective local practice: A pragmatic framework for improving culturally competent practice in psychology. *Professional Psychology: Research and Practice, 49*(2), 142.

Sawyer, W., & Wagner, P. (2020). *Mass incarceration: The whole pie 2020* (Vol. 24). Prison Policy Initiative.

Scharff, A., Roberson, K., Sutherland, M. E., & Boswell, J. F. (2021). Black therapists working with Black clients: Intervention use and caseload preferences. *Practice Innovations, 6*(2), 77.

Schwarz, A. (2011, July 19). School discipline study raises new questions. *The New York Times.* www.nytimes.com/2011/07/19/education/19discipline.html

Sickmund, M., Sladky, T. J., Puzzanchera, C., & Kang, W. (2021). Easy access to the census of juveniles in residential placement. National Center for Juvenile Justice. www.ojjdp.gov/ojstatbb/ezacjrp

Skiba, R. J., Arredondo, M. I., & Williams, N. T. (2014). More than a metaphor: The contribution of exclusionary discipline to a school-to-prison pipeline. *Equity & Excellence in Education, 47*, 546–564.

Skiba, R. J., Chung, C. G., Trachok, M., Baker, T. L., Sheya, A., & Hughes, R. L. (2014). Parsing disciplinary disproportionality: Contributions of infraction, student, and school characteristics to out-of-school suspension and expulsion. *American Educational Research Journal, 51*(4), 640–670.

Skiba, R. J., Horner, R. H., Chung, C.-G., Rausch, M. K., May, S. L., & Tobin, T. (2011). Race is not neutral: A national investigation of African American and Latino disproportionality in school discipline. *School Psychology Review, 40*, 85–107.

Skiba, R. J., Michael, R. S., Nardo, A. C., & Peterson, R. L. (2002). The color of discipline: Sources of racial and gender disproportionality in school punishment. *Urban Review, 34*, 317–342.

Smith, D., Ortiz, N. A., Blake, J. J., Marchbanks, M., Unni, A., & Peguero, A. A. (2021). Tipping point: Effect of the number of in-school suspensions on academic failure. *Contemporary School Psychology, 25*, 466–475.

Smith, W. H. (2010). *The impact of racial trauma on African Americans.* African American Men and Boys Advisory Board.

Spiegelman, M. (2020). Race and ethnicity of public school teachers and their students. Data Point. NCES 2020-103. *National Center for Education Statistics.*

Startz, D. (2020, January). *The achievement gap in education: Racial segregation versus segregation by poverty.* Brookings. *www.brookings.edu/articles/the-achievement-gap-in-education-racial-segregation-versus-segregation-by-poverty*

Steele, J. M., & Newton, C. S. (2022). Culturally adapted cognitive behavioral therapy as a model to address internalized racism among African American clients. *Journal of Mental Health Counseling, 44*(2), 98–116.

Stern, A. (2020). Forced sterilization policies in the U.S. targeted minorities and those with disabilities—And lasted into the 21st century. *Institute for Healthcare Policy and Innovation, University of Michigan.*

Substance Abuse and Mental Health Services Administration, Center for Behavioral Health Statistics and Quality. (2022). *National survey on drug use and health: African Americans 2022* (Document NSDUH-2022).

Sue, D. W., Capodilupo, C. M., Torino, G. C., Bucceri, J. M., Holder, A., Nadal, K. L., & Esquilin, M. (2007). Racial microaggressions in everyday life: Implications for clinical practice. *American Psychologist, 62*(4), 271.

Sue, S. (1999). Science, ethnicity, and bias: Where have we gone wrong? *American Psychologist, 54*(12), 1070.

Tenenbaum H. R., & Ruck, M. D. (2007). Are teachers' expectations different for racial minority than for European American students? A meta-analysis. *Journal of Educational Psychology, 99,* 253–273.

Tervalon, M., & Murray-Garcia, J. (1998). Cultural humility versus cultural competence: A critical distinction in defining physician training outcomes in multicultural education. *Journal of Health Care for the Poor and Underserved, 9*(2), 117–125.

Trent, M., Dooley, D. G., Dougé, J., Cavanaugh, R. M., Lacroix, A. E., Fanburg, J., & Wallace, S. B. (2019). The impact of racism on child and adolescent health. *Pediatrics, 144*(2).

Turner, N., Hastings, J. F., & Neighbors, H. W. (2019). Mental health care treatment seeking among African Americans and Caribbean Blacks: What is the role of religiosity/spirituality? *Aging & Mental Health, 23*(7), 905–911.

Tyson, K. (2002). Weighing in: Elementary-age students and the debate on attitudes toward school among Black students. *Social Forces, 80,* 1157–1189.

U.S. Department of Education. (2020, September 22). Race and ethnicity of public school teachers and their students. *https://nces.ed.gov/pubsearch/pubsinfo.asp?pubid=2020103*

U.S. Department of Education (USDOE)–Office for Civil Rights. (2016). 2013–14 Civil rights data collection: A first look (p. 13).

Upshaw, N. C., Lewis, D. E., Jr., & Nelson, A. L. (2020). Cultural humility in action: Reflective and process-oriented supervision with Black trainees. *Training and Education in Professional Psychology, 14*(4), 277.

Wallace, J. M., Goodkind, S., Wallace, C. M., & Bachman, J. G. (2008). Racial, ethnic, and gender differences in school discipline among U.S. high school students: 1991–2005. *Negro Educational Review, 59*(1–2), 47–62.

Wang, M., & Del Toro, J. (2021). The longitudinal inter-relations between school discipline and academic performance: Examining the role of school climate. *American Psychologist, 75*, 173–185.

Washington, H. A. (2006). *Medical apartheid: The dark history of medical experimentation on Black Americans from colonial times to the present*. Doubleday.

Watts, R. (2021, June 11). 5 Strategies to help black students feel at home in school. *www.edutopia.org/article/5-strategies-help-black-students-feel-home-school*

Weissman, M., Cregor, M., Center, S. P. L., & Gainsborough, A. J. (2008). The right to education in the juvenile and criminal justice systems in the United States. *Dignity in Schools Campaign*.

White, J. (1970). Toward a Black psychology. *Ebony, 25*(11), 44–45.

Will, M. (2020, July 8). Future teachers mistake black students as "angry" more than white students, study shows. *Education Week*. www.edweek.org/leadership/future-teachers-mistake-black-students-as-angry-more-than-white-students-study-shows/2020/07

Winfrey, O., & Perry, B. (2021). *What happened to you?: Conversations on trauma, resilience, and healing*. Boxtree.

Winslade, J., & Williams, M. (2017). Re-entry conversations: A restorative narrative practice for student reintegration. *Narrative and Conflict: Explorations in Theory and Practice, 6*(1), 22–42.

WNYC. (2015, November 11). School discipline: From corporal punishment to mediation. *The Takeaway*. www.wnyc.org/story/school-discipline-corporal-punishment-mediation

Worrell, F. C., & Dixson, D. D. (2020). Diversity and gifted education. In J. A. Plucker & C. M. Callahan (Eds.), *Critical issues and practices in gifted education—A survey of current research on giftedness and talent development* (3rd ed., pp. 169–184). Routledge.

X, M. (1964). Malcolm X's speech at the Founding Rally of the Organization of Afro-American Unity. www.blackpast.org/african-american-history/speeches-african-american-history/1964-malcolm-x-s-speech-founding-rally-organization-afro-american-unity

Yoon, S. Y., & Gentry, M. (2009). Racial and ethnic representation in gifted programs: Current status of and implications for gifted Asian American students. *Gifted Child Quarterly, 53*(2), 121–136.

Young, J. L., & Butler, B. R. (2018). A student saved is not a dollar earned: A meta-analysis of school disparities in discipline practice toward Black children. *Taboo: The Journal of Culture and Education, 17*(4), 6.

Zane, S. N., & Pupo, J. A. (2021). Disproportionate minority contact in the juvenile justice system: A systematic review and meta-analysis. *Justice Quarterly, 38*(7), 1–26.

Zill, N., & Wilcox, W. (2019, November 19). The black and white divide in suspension: What is the role of the family. *Institute for Family Studies.* https://ifstudies.org/blog/the-black-white-divide-in-suspensions-what-is-the-role-of-family

Index

Note. Bold in a page number indicates a Glossary term.

Acceptance, 133–134
Achievement gap, 64, 68–70, **163**. *See also* School settings
Acknowledgement, 133–134, 161
ADDRESSING framework, 54–56, 57. *See also* Culturally responsive supervision; Identity
Adverse childhood experience (ACE), 5–8
Advocacy, 117–118, 122–123, 160
Affirmation
    individual healing from racial trauma and, 133–134, 161
    racial socialization and, 109–110
    racial trauma and, 132
African/Black psychology, 82, 130–132, **163**
Alcohol use, 94
Anger, 133, 140–141, 157
Association of Black Psychologists (ABPsi), 141–142
Assumptions, 113–114

B

Barriers to treatment. *See also* Treatment
    availability of and options for services and, 36
    facilitators for treatment seeking and, 39–42
    overview, 32–35, 42
    process of finding a therapist and, 33–34, 35
    stigma of seeking treatment and, 36–39
Bias. *See also* Explicit bias; Hidden spot; Implicit bias
    building racial competency skills and, 122
    culturally responsive supervision and, 51–52, 57
    discipline practices in school settings and, 70–72
    explicit bias, 16–17, 165
    implicit bias, 16–17, 166
    parenting and, 108, 110–111, 113
    systemic issues and, 9–11

Black Lives Matter (BLM), 97, **164**
Black/African psychology, 82, 130–132, **163**
Black/white achievement gap. *See* Achievement gap
Blind spot. *See* Hidden spot
Blue Lives Matter, 97, **164**
Boundaries, 149
Brain development, 5
Brave spaces, creating, 57–58, 99–100
Burnout, 87, 149–155, 161–162, **164**

C

Called in, 103, **164**
Called out, 103, **164**
Caregiving system, 112. *See also* Parenting
Child-rearing. *See* Parenting
Civil rights, 88, 109, 117, **164**
Clinicians. *See also* Supervision; Vicarious racial trauma; Vicarious trauma
  advocacy role of, 117–118
  clinician's racial identity and, 11–12
  community-level healing, 141–143
  consultant role of, 96–103, 157
  demographics of, 147
  discussing race and, 151–155
  facilitators for treatment seeking and, 41–42
  healing from racial trauma and, 132–144, 157–158
  interventions in school settings and, 76–83
  joining with and supporting parents, 111–112
  organizations and, 155–157, 158
  preparing to work with parents and children and, 110–111
  process of finding a therapist and, 33–34, 35, 42, 160
  psychological health of, 149–155, 161–162
  racial trauma and, 145–149
  reflective local practice (RLP) and, 19–21, 51–52
  roles of, 96–103, 117–118, 157, 159–162
  school settings and, 65–68, 69–70
  supporting African American parents and, 112–118, 122–123
  techniques for working with Black law enforcement officers, 91–95
  training and, 16–17
Code switching, 139, **164**
Cognitive restructuring, 24–28
Cognitive-behavioral therapy (CBT), 24–30. *See also* Treatment
Community settings, 141–143. *See also* Law enforcement settings; School settings
Complex trauma, 7, **165**. *See also* Psychological trauma; Trauma
Confidence, 109–110
Consultant role, 96–103, 157. *See also* Clinicians
Continuing education, 160. *See also* Training
Coping
  clinicians' experience of racial trauma and, 149
  helping clients develop or access coping skills, 119–121, 143–144
  overview, 132
  racial socialization and, 109–110
  techniques for working with Black law enforcement officers, 91–95
Counteract devaluation, 133, 139–140
COVID-19 pandemic, 34, 46, 93–94
Creating a Respectful and Open World for Natural Hair (CROWN) Act, 67–68, **165**
Creating space for race
  discussing race in therapy and, 151–155
  individual healing from racial trauma and, 133, 134–135, 161
  organizations and, 155–157
Criminal justice system. *See* Law enforcement settings; School-to-prison pipeline
Cultural competence
  culturally responsive supervision and, 58
  definition, **165**
  facilitators for treatment seeking and, 40
  overview, 17–18, 30
  reflective local practice (RLP) and, 19–21
  role of clinicians in supporting African American parents and, 113–114
  supervision and, 47–50
Cultural humility
  culturally responsive supervision and, 58
  definition, **165**

facilitators for treatment seeking and, 40
improving supervisory skills and, 56–57
organizations and, 157
overview, 17–18, 30
supervision and, 47–52
Cultural pride, 108–109, 114
Culturally responsive instruction, 65, 118
Culturally responsive supervision. *See also* Supervision; Teachers
clinicians' experience of racial trauma and, 148–149
cultural humility and, 50–52
identity and, 54–56
improving supervisory skills and, 56–58
overview, 48–49, 53–56, 58–59
Culture, departmental, 96–103

D

Department culture, 96–103
Depression, 9–10, 33–34
Devaluation, 92, 133, 138–140
Diagnosis
facilitators for treatment seeking and, 41
historical context of, 18–19
overview, 9–10, 15
stigma of seeking treatment and, 36–39
Diagnostic and Statistical Manual of Mental Disorders, Fifth Edition (DSM-5), 73
Discipline practices in school settings, 70–72, 76–83. *See also* School settings
Discrimination
advocacy role of clinicians and, 117–118
building racial competency skills and, 122
definition, **165**
facilitators for treatment seeking and, 40
impact of on treatment, 16–17, 42
overview, 8
parenting and, 108, 109–110, 113
racial socialization and, 109–110
reflective local practice (RLP) and, 20
role of clinicians in supporting African American parents and, 113
in school settings, 67–69
trauma-focused cognitive-behavioral therapy and, 22–24
Drug use, 94

E

Educational environments. *See* School settings
Emotional Emancipation Circles (EECs), 141–142
Empowerment, 141–142
Engaging, Managing, and Bonding through race (EMBrace) model, 119–121
Environmental stressors, 6–7, 40. *See also* Law enforcement settings; School settings
Equity
definition, **165**
organizations and, 155–157
school settings and, 65
Eurocentric psychology, 131
Explicit bias, 16–17, **165**. *See also* Bias
Externalized devaluation, 133, 138–139

F

Facilitators for treatment seeking, 39–42. *See also* Treatment
Faith, 119–121, 142–143
Fit between clinician and client. *See* Clinicians; Therapeutic alliance

G

Gifted education programs, 76–77. *See also* School settings

H

Hair "norms," 67–68
Healing
as a community, 141–143
individual healing from racial trauma and, 132–141
organizations and, 155–157
overview, 132, 143–144
Health care system, 10
Healthy cultural suspicion, 93–94, 113

Hidden spot. *See also* Bias
  culturally responsive supervision and, 48–49, 51–52
  definition, **165**
  preparing to work with parents and children and, 110–111
Hot spots, 51. *See also* Bias
Humility. *See* Cultural humility

I

Identity. *See also* Racial identity
  culturally responsive supervision and, 54–56, 58
  person-centered language and, 9
  preparing to work with parents and children and, 110–111
  racially competent teaching and, 82–83
  reflective local practice (RLP) and, 19–21
  techniques for working with Black law enforcement officers, 93
Implicit bias, 16–17, **166**. *See also* Bias
Institutionalized racism, 86. *See also* Racism
Insurance, 41–42
Integrative approach to treatment, 28–30, 31. *See also* Treatment
Internalized devaluation, 92
Internalized racism, 112, **166**. *See also* Racial identity; Racism
Interpersonal interventions, 28–30. *See also* Treatment
Intersectionality, 50
Interventions, 76–83. *See also* Treatment

L

Law enforcement settings. *See also* School-to-prison pipeline
  overview, 85–88, 103–104, 160–161
  techniques for working with Black officers, 91–95
  working with agencies after racialized trauma, 96–103
  working with individual officers, 88–91
Learning disabilities, 76

M

Macroassaults, 95, 137–138, **166**. *See also* Microaggressions
Management commitment sessions, 156–157
Mandatory training, 98–100. *See also* Training
Marginalization, 57–58
Mass incarceration, 72–75. *See also* Criminal justice system
Mediation, 81–82
Mental health diagnosis, 9–10, 36–39. *See also* Diagnosis
Mental illness, 33–34
Microaggressions. *See also* Macroassaults
  culturally responsive supervision and, 49–50, 53–54
  definition, **166**
  improving supervisory skills and, 56–57
  naming racial experiences and, 137–138
  organizations and, 155
  overview, 8
Mood disorders, 9–10
Motivational interviewing (MI), 89–90, **166**
Multicultural supervision. *See* Culturally responsive supervision; Supervision
Murders of Black people. *See also* Racial trauma
  Brown, Michael, 85–86
  Castile, Philando, 90–91
  Floyd, George, 34, 35, 145
  Garner, Eric, 85–86
  overview, 34, 35, 145–146
  supervision and, 46
  Taylor, Breonna, 34
  working with individual law-enforcement officers and, 90–91

N

Naming racial experiences, 133, 137–138, 161
Neurobiological impact, 5–8

O

Obsessive–compulsive disorder (OCD), 9–10
Oppression, racial. *See* Racial oppression
Organizations, 155–157, 158

P

Parenting
   advocacy role of clinicians and, 117–118
   building coping skills and, 119–121
   building racial competency skills, 121–122
   interventions in school settings and, 78–80
   joining with and supporting parents, 111–112
   preparing to work with parents and children and, 110–111
   providing psychoeducation and, 118–119
   racial socialization and, 108–110, 111–112, 122–123
   role of clinicians in supporting African American parents and, 112–118, 122–123, 161
P.E.A.C.E. (Positive Energy Activates Constant Elevation) groups, 156
Peer consultation groups, 157
Peer supervision, 160. *See also* Supervision
Person-centered language, 8–9. *See also* Terminology
Physiological symptoms, 94
Police officers, 75, 110. *See also* Law enforcement settings
Police-related racial trauma. *See* Law enforcement settings; Murders of Black people; Racial trauma
Political environment, 34–35, 46, 110
Posttraumatic stress disorder (PTSD)
   barriers to treatment and, 34
   definition, **166**
   diagnosis and, 9–10
   law enforcement settings and, 87
   vicarious trauma and, 147
Power, 50
Prejudices, 122
Preparation, 110
Pride, racial, 108–109, 113, 136

Privilege, 12, 50, **167**
Professional development, 83, 84. *See also* Training
Psychodynamic interventions, 28–30. *See also* Treatment
Psychoeducation
   joining with and supporting parents, 111–112
   racial socialization and, 118–119
   trauma-focused cognitive-behavioral therapy and, 22
Psychological symptoms, 94
Psychological trauma, 7, **167**. *See also* Complex trauma; Trauma

R

Race-based traumatic stress. *See also* Trauma
   approaches to care and, 14
   definition, **167**
   overview, 7–8, 15
   person-centered language and, 9
   systemic issues and, 9–11
Racial achievement gap. *See* Achievement gap
Racial identity. *See also* Identity
   clinicians' racial identity and, 11–12
   culturally responsive supervision and, 50–52, 54–56, 58
   definition, **167**
   individual healing from racial trauma and, 132–141
   internalized racism and, 112
   preparing to work with parents and children and, 110–111
   racially competent teaching and, 82–83
   techniques for working with Black law enforcement officers, 93
   trauma-focused cognitive-behavioral therapy and, 23–24
Racial microaggressions, 49–50. *See also* Microaggressions
Racial oppression
   culturally responsive supervision and, 57–58
   definition, **167**
   naming racial experiences and, 137–138

Racial pride, 108–109, 113, 136
Racial socialization
  building coping skills and, 119–121
  building racial competency skills, 121–122
  joining with and supporting parents, 111–112
  overview, 108–110, 122–123
  providing psychoeducation and, 118–119
  role of clinicians in supporting African American parents and, 112–118
  trauma-focused cognitive-behavioral therapy and, 22
Racial Socialization Competency Scale (RaSCS), 121–122
Racial storytelling, 133, 135–136
Racial trauma. *See also* Trauma; Vicarious racial trauma
  barriers to treatment and, 35
  clinicians' experience of, 11–12, 145–149, 161–162
  definition, **167**
  example of case conceptualization through a lens of, 12–14
  facilitators for treatment seeking and, 40
  individual healing from, 132–141
  law enforcement settings and, 86–87, 91–104
  naming racial experiences and, 137–138
  overview, 8, 15, 159–160
  person-centered language and, 9
  psychological health of clinicians and, 149–155
  school settings and, 65–66, 68–70
  school-to-prison pipeline and, 73
  treatment and, 127–132, 143–144
Racially competent teaching, 82–83, 84. *See also* School settings; Teachers
Racism. *See also* Systemic factors
  advocacy role of clinicians and, 117–118
  building racial competency skills and, 122
  clinicians' experience of, 146–147
  definition, **167**
  facilitators for treatment seeking and, 40
  impact of on treatment, 16–17, 42
  institutionalized racism, 86
  internalized racism, 112, **166**
  law enforcement settings and, 86
  naming racial experiences and, 137–138
  overview, 7, 8, 15

  parenting and, 108, 113
  person-centered language and, 9
  reflective local practice (RLP) and, 20
  structural racism, 68, **168**
  systemic issues and, 9–11
  trauma-focused cognitive-behavioral therapy and, 22–24
Rage, rechanneling, 133, 140–141
Rapport, 67
Reflective local practice (RLP)
  culturally responsive supervision and, 51–52, 58
  definition, **167**
  overview, 19–21, 30–31
  preparing to work with parents and children and, 111
  role of clinicians in supporting African American parents and, 114
Reflectiveness, 50–52, 57. *See also* Reflective local practice (RLP)
Relationships, 98
Religious practices, 119–121, 142–143
Resilience, 109–110
Resistance, 117–118
Responsiveness, 50–52
Restorative protocols, 77–80

S

Sankofa Violence Prevention Program, 81–82
Sawubona Healing Circles, 142–143
Schizophrenia, 9–10
School settings. *See also* Achievement gap
  clinicians in, 65–68, 69–70
  discipline practices and, 70–72
  interventions and, 76–83
  overview, 63–64, 83–84, 160
  race-based bias and, 10
  racial trauma and, 68–70
  racially competent teaching and, 82–83
  school-to-prison pipeline and, 72–75
  supporting African American parents and, 112–118
  teacher demographics, 64–65
School-to-prison pipeline, 64, 72–75, 160, **168**. *See also* School settings
Self-awareness, 56–57

Self-care
   clinicians' experience of racial trauma and, 149, 157
   definition, **168**
   psychological health of clinicians and, 149–155, 161–162
Self-reflection
   culturally responsive supervision and, 49
   improving supervisory skills and, 57
   preparing to work with parents and children and, 110–111
   reflective local practice (RLP) and, 19–21
Self-worth
   interventions in school settings and, 80
   parenting and, 108
   racial socialization and, 109–110
Shootings of Black people. *See* Murders of Black people; Racial trauma
Socialization, racial. *See* Racial socialization
Sociopolitical factors, 34–35, 46, 110
Soft spots, 52. *See also* Bias
Space for race
   discussing race in therapy and, 151–155
   individual healing from racial trauma and, 133, 134–135, 161
   organizations and, 155–157
Special education services, 76. *See also* School settings
Spiritual practices, 119–121, 142–143
Stigmatization
   barriers to treatment and, 36–39
   definition, **168**
   diagnosis and, 10
   treatment and, 16–17
Stress. *See also* Toxic stress
   impact of, 5
   overview, 15
   school settings and, 69
   techniques for working with Black law enforcement officers, 93–96
Structural racism, 68, **168**. *See also* Racism
Substance use, 94
Supervision. *See also* Clinicians; Culturally responsive supervision
   clinicians' experience of racial trauma and, 148–149
   cultural competence and cultural humility and, 47–52
   improving supervisory skills and, 56–58
   overview, 43–45, 53–56
   peer supervision, 160
   role of a supervisor and, 45–47
Suspension. *See* Discipline practices in school settings; School settings
Suspicion, 93–94, 113
Systemic factors
   barriers to treatment and, 33–34
   clinicians' experience of racial trauma and, 158
   overview, 9–11
   school-to-prison pipeline and, 73
   trauma-focused cognitive-behavioral therapy and, 23
Systemic racism. *See also* Racism
   systemic racism, 86

T

The Talk, 108–109, 110. *See also* Parenting; Racial socialization
Teachers. *See also* School settings
   advocacy role of clinicians and, 118
   clinicians in school settings and, 66
   overview, 64–65, 83–84
   racial socialization and, 110
   racially competent teaching and, 82–83
Terminology
   hidden spot, 48*n*
   naming racial experiences and, 137–138, 161
   overview, 8–9
   working with law enforcement agencies after racialized trauma, 101
Therapeutic alliance. *See also* Clinicians; Treatment
   advocacy role of clinicians and, 117–118
   discussing race and, 151–155
   overview, 33–34
   process of finding a therapist and, 35
   role of clinicians in supporting African American parents and, 117–118
Therapists. *See* Clinicians
Time, narrowed sense of, 94–95
Toxic stress, 5–8, **168**. *See also* Stress
Training
   clinicians in school settings and, 66
   culturally responsive supervision and, 48, 50–51, 58–59

Training (cont.)
  facilitators for treatment seeking and, 39
  improving supervisory skills and, 56–58
  organizations and, 155–157
  overview, 30–31
  process of finding a therapist and, 35
  racially competent teaching and, 83, 84
  reflective local practice (RLP) and, 11–12, 19–20
  role of a supervisor and, 45–47
  teacher preparation programs and, 65
  working with law enforcement agencies after racialized trauma, 96–103
Trauma. *See also* Complex trauma; Psychological trauma; Race-based traumatic stress; Racial trauma
  definition, **168**
  impact of, 5
  neurobiological impact of, 5–8
  overview, 15
Trauma-focused cognitive-behavioral therapy (TF-CBT), 22–24. *See also* Treatment
Trauma-informed care. *See also* Treatment
  overview, 130–131
  race-based traumatic stress and, 11
  racially competent teaching and, 82–83
  trauma-focused cognitive-behavioral therapy, 22–24
Traumatic stress. *See* Race-based traumatic stress; Trauma
Treatment. *See also* Barriers to treatment
  advocacy role of clinicians and, 117–118
  approaches to care and, 14, 21–30
  availability of and options for, 36
  building coping skills and, 119–121
  building racial competency skills, 121–122
  community-level healing, 141–143
  discipline practices in school settings and, 71–72
  discussing race and, 151–155
  facilitators for treatment seeking and, 39–42
  healing from racial trauma and, 141–144
  historical context of, 18–19
  individual healing from racial trauma and, 132–141
  integration of techniques, 28–30
  law enforcement settings and, 88–95, 96–103
  organizations and, 155–157
  overview, 159–162
  parenting and, 110–118
  process of finding a therapist and, 33–34, 42, 160
  race-based bias and, 9–11
  racial trauma and, 127–132
  reflective local practice (RLP) and, 19–21
Treatment facilitators, 39–42. *See also* Treatment
Treatment-resistant populations, 88–91

V

Validation
  individual healing from racial trauma and, 133, 136–137
  motivational interviewing and, 89–90
  psychoeducation and, 119
Vicarious racial trauma, 146–150, 155, **168**. *See also* Clinicians; Racial trauma; Vicarious trauma
Vicarious trauma. *See also* Clinicians; Racial trauma; Trauma; Vicarious racial trauma
  clinicians' experience of, 146–149, 161–162
  definition, **168**
  law enforcement settings and, 87, 93–96
  overview, 7–8, 68–69
  psychological health of clinicians and, 149–155
Vigilance, 93–94
Voluntary training, 98–100. *See also* Training

www.ingramcontent.com/pod-product-compliance
Ingram Content Group UK Ltd.
Pitfield, Milton Keynes, MK11 3LW, UK
UKHW032012110225
454920UK00001B/17